W9-AAV-355

THIRD EDITION

ESSAYS

that will get you into

Medical School

Adrienne Dowhan, Chris Dowhan, and Dan Kaufman

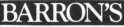

© Copyright 2009, 2003, 1998 by Daniel Kaufman

All rights reserved. No part of this publication may be reproduced or distributed in any form or by any means without the written permission of the copyright owner.

All inquiries should be addressed to:
Barron's Educational Series, Inc.
250 Wireless Boulevard
Hauppauge, NY 11788
www.barronseduc.com

Library of Congress Catalog Card No. 2009003709

ISBN-13: 978-0-7641-4227-7
ISBN-10: 0-7641-4227-5

Library of Congress Cataloging-in-Publication Data
Dowhan, Adrienne.
   Essays that will get you into medical school / Adrienne Dowhan,
Chris Dowhan, Daniel Kaufman.—3rd ed.
      p.   cm.
   Includes index.
   ISBN-13: 978-0-7641-4227-7
   ISBN-10: 0-7641-4227-5
   1. Medical colleges—United States—Admission.   2. Exposition (Rhetoric)
3. Essay—Authorship.   4. Medical colleges—United States—Entrance
requirements.   I. Dowhan, Chris.   II. Kaufman, Daniel, 1968–   III. Title.
   R838.4.D69   2009
   610.71'173—dc22

                                                      2009003709

Printed in the United States of America
9 8 7 6 5

Contents

ACKNOWLEDGMENTS v
INTRODUCTION vii
A NOTE ABOUT PLAGIARISM ix

PART ONE
Applying to Medical School   1

Pre-med Courses 2
MCAT 2
AMCAS 3
Secondary Applications 5
Letters of Recommendation 5
The Interview 5
A Note About Fees 5

PART TWO
Preparing to Write the Essay   7

ASSESS YOUR AUDIENCE 9
Knowing Your Audience 10
What the Admissions Committee Is Looking For 11
What the Admissions Committee Is Tired of Reading 17
Get Feedback 19

GATHER YOUR MATERIAL 20
Seek Inspiration Through Examples 21
Creative Writing Exercises 21
Assess Yourself 23
Before You Move On 25

DEVELOP A STRATEGY 26
Identify Your Themes 27
Strategic Tips 36
An Alternative Approach 39

PART THREE
Writing the Essay   41

AT LAST, WRITE! 43
Creating an Outline 44
Incorporating the Narrative 48
Structuring the Paragraphs 49
Creating Effective Transitions 50
Choosing the Right Words 50
Composing Proper Sentences 51

Writing Introductions and Conclusions 52
Taking a Break 56

MAKE IT PERFECT **57**
Revise 57
The Hunt for Red Flags 60
Proofread 60
Read Out Loud 61
Get Feedback 61

PART FOUR
The Interview   63

PREPARING FOR THE INTERVIEW **65**
Types of Interviews 66
Tips for Interviewing Successfully 66
Notes About Etiquette 69

COMMON INTERVIEW QUESTIONS **71**
Questions Interviewers Will Ask You 72
Questions You Can Ask Interviewers 78

PART FIVE
Compilation of AMCAS Personal Statements   81

ESSAY INDEX 168
INDEX 171

Acknowledgments

The authors of this book are all part of an Internet-based company called IvyEssays.com. Since its creation in 1996, IvyEssays' goal has been to help students gain admission to leading colleges and graduate schools by providing them with a variety of resources such as examples of previously successful essays and professional editing services.

We owe our sincere thanks to two groups of people. First there are all the students who have permitted us to publish their admissions essays so they might illuminate the way for future rounds of hopeful applicants. Second, there is the team of IvyEssays' contributors—past and present admissions officers and professional writers who together have logged more than 50 years of admissions experience. This series would not have been possible without the assistance of those cited below.

Ellen M. Watts has worked in graduate admissions for nine years and is currently the Director of Admissions and Student Affairs at Columbia University School of Dental and Oral Surgery, where she screens more than 2000 applications annually. In addition, she serves as an independent admissions counselor, specializing in interview skills workshops.

Amy Yerkes was an instructor at the University of Maryland School of Medicine where she taught a course designed to increase the writing skills of prospective medical students for the Office of Minority Student Affairs. She has also taught at the University of Pennsylvania and is currently Assistant to the Dean at Johns Hopkins University School of Continuing Studies and a lecturer at Western Maryland College.

Joanna Henderson was Director of Graduate Admissions responsible for M.B.A. programs at Babson for four years and the Dean of Admissions at Colby-Sawyer College for five years. She is presently Director of the New England Admissions Office at Marietta College in Ohio and is an advisor/consultant for Stanley Kaplan Educational Center. She is the author of ZINGERS! *Creating Achievements from Ordinary Experiences,* published in 1988.

Miriam Ruth Albert is an assistant professor of Legal and Ethical studies at Fordham University Schools of Business. She was a Legal Methods professor and Associate Director of Admissions at Widener University School of Law where she counseled prospective applicants and evaluated more than 400 applications. She also taught an LSAT preparation course for Stanley Kaplan Educational Center.

Amy Engle worked at the Hofstra University School of Law for seven years and served there as Assistant Dean of Admissions.

Helen LaFave is an independent consultant who counsels prospective students through all stages of the admissions process. She has also served as Senior Programs Officer and Recruitment Program Officer at Columbia University where she helped numerous students through extensive graduate school application processes.

Thomas Vance Sturgeon has more than eight years experience in the admissions process as Associate Director of Admissions at Duke University and Assistant Director of Admissions at Guilford College. He is currently the Director of Admissions at the South Carolina School for Science and Mathematics. Mr. Sturgeon is a widely published author and lecturer on the subject of college admissions, and has been quoted in *Money Magazine's Guide to Colleges* and published in the *Journal of College Admissions*.

Marcy Whaley is the former Associate Director of Admissions at the California Institute of Technology and Assistant Dean of Admissions at Illinois Institute of Technology. She has more than a decade of experience in college admissions and today is an independent admissions consultant and freelance technical writer.

Scott Anderson is Associate Director of Admissions at Cornell University. Mr. Anderson's past experience includes the position of Assistant Director of Admissions at Vassar College, and he has been on the admissions staffs at the University of Vermont, St. Michael's College, and the University of Virginia.

Patricia M. Soares is an independent educational consultant for underprivileged youth with years of experience as an admissions officer. She has been Assistant Director of Admissions at Connecticut College and an admissions officer at Rhode Island College.

IvyEssays was founded based on the belief that some people have more access than others to the resources and information that improve one's chances of getting into the top schools. While admissions officers do their best to take these disparities into account, it is up to students to equip themselves for the application process to the best of their abilities. IvyEssays hopes that its services can help level the admissions playing field by providing resources that might otherwise be available only to the privileged. Good luck and good writing!

Introduction

So you want to go to medical school?

Whether you are still researching the application process, are looking for inspiration for the daunting essay, or are ready to put your words on paper, this book is designed to give you all the tools you will need. In these pages you will discover what a vital role the essay plays in the application process, you will find over 35 essays that were actually accepted at some of the nation's top medical schools, and you will be given tools that will allow you to write stellar essays of your own and to ultimately sail through the interview that your essay WILL help you secure.

What's in this book?

In our 3rd edition of *Essays That Will Get You into Medical School* we have added a section that lays out the process of applying to medical school, in sequential steps with some important tips and facts about each. The bulk of the book still focuses, of course, on the essay and we have included comments after each essay that reveal its strengths as well as how it could have been improved. These essays will prove invaluable to you as you search for ideas and inspiration for your own essays and probably struggle (who doesn't?) with concerns of how your writing skills and breadth of experiences stack up to the rest of the applicant pool. Finally, we walk you through the interview process, providing questions that admissions officers have shared with us, and prepare you to answer them honestly and wisely.

Why is the personal statement widely considered the most important part of your application?

First, it is likely the only part of the application that you have control over. Second, without a personal statement that makes the application committee find you interesting enough to want to know you better, the coveted interview may never happen.

So consider this in the writing process: Everything you have done up to now is completed—past tense. You couldn't change it if you wanted to, so stop worrying about it. The personal statement lies ahead—treat it as if it is the only thing that matters.

Imagine that the only thing an admissions committee would ever see is your essay. One to two pages, double-spaced, are all they would have to make a decision that will change the rest of your life. As one admissions officer stated:

Students do have a lot of control. They may feel powerless in the face of the medical application process, but what they show us in the essay and interview is up to them. They shouldn't underestimate the importance of this.

The personal statement and the interview allow you to humanize yourself.

Think of your personal statement as the face of your application. An application without an essay is a statistic; it's just another faceless person in a crowd.

As a member of the admissions committee at Harvard Medical School and a premedical advisor at Harvard College, I realize that the personal statement is the only way that an admissions committee member can get to know an applicant and, therefore, the essay should be written and rewritten, read and proofread, countless times.

An application with a poorly written essay doesn't give admissions officers the opportunity to care. It's basic psychology: Make them feel that they know you, and it will be harder for them to reject you. Make them know you and like you, and they might accept you despite weakness in other areas.

The personal statement—and the interview provide you with an opportunity to showcase your social skills.

The personal statement is the most misunderstood portion of the medical application. Students approach it with fear, and never feel they have tackled it from the proper angle, which is a mistake. Each student should look upon this section as an opportunity to humanize their otherwise academic-emphasized application folder.

Not only will humanizing yourself through the essay make you more memorable to the admissions committee, but the committee is also aware that strong social skills and a likeable character are important qualities in a doctor.

Understanding the importance of the personal statement and the interview is a necessary first step toward perfecting your medical school application, but that knowledge alone won't do you much good. In fact, it could even hurt your efforts if it only makes you nervous. So, if this whole application process has you perspiring, you can relax now. Taking the process seriously is the first step. We're here to help you get through the rest. Let's get started!

A Note About Plagiarism

Throughout this book, we have emphasized the need for honest, personal application essays. To submit anything else to the schools you are applying to is not only stupid—it's illegal.

If you do borrow material from other sources, be sure to credit it properly. If you are not careful about this, you may hurt your chances of getting into a particular school. To purposely avoid giving credit where credit is due is to court disaster.

An admissions officer was once quoted as saying, "After fifteen years of reading hundreds of essays a year, you develop an amazing ability to see straight through the bull." This is also true of detecting plagiarism. Admissions officers do read hundreds of essays every year. In doing so, they have developed a sense of whether or not the author of the essay is being honest. Although it may sound impossible, these admissions officers also tend to remember many of the essays that they read. If it is discovered that you have "borrowed" someone else's essay, you will undoubtedly be denied admission.

You owe it to yourself to be honest, forthright, and sincere.

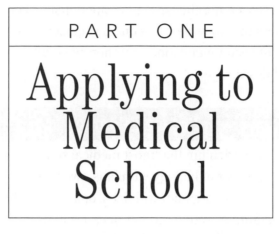

PART ONE

Applying to Medical School

Highlights

- Applying to medical school is a 5-step process.
  1. Completing pre-med courses
  2. Taking the MCAT
  3. Completing the AMCAS application
  4. Filling out secondary applications for individual schools
  5. Requesting letters of recommendation
- You will receive invitations to interview by schools that are considering accepting you.
- The Fee Assistance Program (FAP) developed by the AAMC can offset the exorbitant cost of applying to medical school.

You may not have known it then, but the process of applying to medical school began many years ago. It may have begun with a childhood experience that instilled in you a desire to help others, or maybe it began with the frog you dissected in high school that sparked your fascination with living creatures, how they are composed and how they function. It continued with each extracurricular activity, every job experience, and each research project. It was enhanced with every honor and award you received. It began long ago because though you may not have realized it then, you are now being asked to recall each and every experience that will demonstrate you are ready for medical school both academically and emotionally. It may seem daunting but think of it this way—most of the work is already done. What lies ahead is a standardized test, a comprehensive application that will include all college transcripts and your personal statement, secondary applications based on the schools you select, letters of recommendation and then hopefully, the coveted interview. So let's break it all down.

Pre-med Courses

There is a general curriculum that most medical schools require before matriculation. These are one year of biology with labs, two years of chemistry (one year of inorganic and one year of organic) with labs, one year of physics, one year of calculus, and many institutions require a year of expository writing. Harvard Medical School, for example, states that writing is an important skill both for the study and practice of medicine. They will consider any nonscience courses that involved substantial expository writing to fulfill the writing requirement.

Harvard goes on to say, as do many institutions, that while satisfactory completion of the required science and mathematics courses is expected, they like to see at least 16 hours completed in literature, languages, the arts, humanities, and the social sciences. They further recommend honors courses and independent study and/or research. And, of course, computer proficiency is also expected.

It is important to note that while strong performances in the sciences is expected from all applicants, most admissions committees admire students who can demonstrate a well-rounded education through both their course work and their extracurricular activities. So if you didn't major in a science, but have still done well in all of the pre-med requirements, don't worry! This could actually earmark your application as unique, rather than weak.

The average GPA as reported by the Association of American Medical Colleges (AAMC) in 2007 hit an all time high. The average GPA across the total applicant pool of 42,315 was 3.49. That was broken down as 3.39 for the Science GPA and 3.62 for the nonscience GPA. For students who actually matriculated, the average GPA was, of course, even higher with a 3.65 GPA total, broken down as 3.59 for science courses and 3.73 for nonscience courses.

MCAT

The Medical College Admissions Test (MCAT) is required by almost all medical schools as part of the application package. It is a standardized test that is mostly multiple-choice. The exam is designed to assess problem solving, critical thinking, writing skills, and knowledge of science concepts and principles prerequisite to the study of medicine. Because of the heavy focus on science concepts, it is highly recommended that all pre-med courses be completed prior to taking the MCAT. Questions are largely based on this prerequisite curriculum. The cost for taking the MCAT for 2007 examinees was $210.

In 2007, the exam consisted of approximately 50 questions each in physical sciences and biological sciences, 40 questions in verbal reasoning, and 2 writing samples. Scores are reported in each of these four categories. Most schools will not accept MCAT scores that are more than three years old.

As of 2007, several changes were made to the MCAT that made it approximately 30% shorter than the 2006 exam. Testing is now computerized; a pencil and paper option is not available. The exam is only offered in English. Total testing time is approximately four and a half hours. The total appointment time for taking the MCAT is about five hours and twenty minutes, which includes optional tutorials and three ten-minute breaks.

For each of the multiple-choice sections, a numeric score is given. Raw scores are scaled, taking into consideration the difficulty of the test questions. Scaled scores range from 1 to 15. Each writing sample is scored twice and the total raw score is the sum of the four individual scores. The numeric score, which ranges from 1 to 6, is converted to an alphabetic scale that ranges from J (the lowest) to T (the highest). The AAMC reported that in 2007, the mean MCAT scores for all medical school applicants was as follows: VR 9, PS 9.2, BS 9.6, WS O. For those who actually matriculated, scores were slightly higher and were reported as follows: VR 9.9, PS 10.3, BS 10.6, WS P.

AMCAS

AMCAS, short for the American Medical College Application Service, is a centralized application service utilized by almost all American medical schools. It is a web-based application that simplifies the process of applying to multiple medical schools by having applicants fill out one comprehensive application that is then forwarded to each school that the applicant indicates in the application. It is a time-consuming process but the web-based system allows you to fill out part of the application, save it, and come back to it at a later time. Changes can be made to the application up to the time that you "certify" it, indicating that it is true and complete. This virtually seals the application, which is now ready for submission. Changes can be made later if proper guidelines outlined by AMCAS are followed. The application will then need to be recertified.

The fee for the AMCAS application as of this publication was $160 for the first school and $30 for each additional school to which an applicant wants the application sent.

The application includes the following sections:

Biographic Information: Information such as name, social security number, mailing address, contact information, economic information and whether or not you would like to be considered for disadvantaged status.

Post-Secondary Experiences: This section allows you to enter any work experiences, extracurricular activities, awards, honors, or publications that you would like the admissions committee to consider. You may enter up to 15 experiences.

Personal Comments: This is where you will paste your essay. We emphasize the word PASTE here because we cannot stress enough how much work and thought should go into this section of your application. In fact, on the application itself you are asked to consider your statement carefully because "admissions committees place SIGNIFICANT weight on this section." It should be approximately one page. Do not type your essay directly into this section of the application. It should be grammatically reviewed and spell-checked until it is perfect. It is interesting to note, however, that a simple text format is best because most of the formatting will be lost when pasted into the application form.

Schools Attended: Here you will enter information about each college you attended. It does not matter if you graduated from each institution. All colleges or universities must be listed even if you only took one course for which you received an incomplete.

Transcript Requests: This section allows you to create and print AMCAS Transcript Request Forms to send to registrars at schools from which official transcripts will be required. It is recommended that you request personal copies of all transcripts in addition to those required for your AMCAS application. Mistakes are not uncommon and this will give you the opportunity to check the transcript for accuracy.

Coursework: In this section, you must enter each course for which you were ever enrolled in any U.S., U.S. Territorial, or Canadian post-secondary institution. This includes courses from which you withdrew, received an incomplete, repeated, failed, are currently enrolled in or expect to enroll in before entering medical school, college-level courses taken in high school, or courses removed from your transcript or GPA as a result of academic bankruptcy, forgiveness, or similar institutional policies.

Certification and Submission: This section includes a final list of questions to which full disclosure is the only policy. Answering "yes" to any of these questions may not hurt your chances of getting into medical school. There is a space left for explanations and a note that "medical schools understand that many individuals learn from the past and emerge stronger as a result." The questions include topics such as institutional action, felonies, and previous matriculation.

*In addition to the sections noted above, AMCAS now allows letters of recommendation to certain schools to be sent in or uploaded from the author.

Secondary Applications

Most medical schools send out secondary applications, otherwise known as supplemental applications, to each student who applies through AMCAS. Many of these schools will not review your application until the secondary application has been returned, complete with letters of recommendation. Other schools will complete a primary screening process before selecting a subset of applicants to which they send the supplemental application. The supplemental application will vary from to school to school but most will require an additional fee ranging from $50-$100, additional essays usually in response to specific questions, and letters of recommendation. It is important to get the secondary applications in as soon as possible because many schools operate on a rolling basis, which means that applications are reviewed as they are received and once they have filled their incoming class with their maximum number of students, you are out of luck.

Letters of Recommendation

All medical schools to which you apply will require letters of recommendation. As previously stated, some schools allow these letters to be uploaded to your AMCAS file. Others will be included with your supplemental applications. Most letters will be sealed—in other words, not reviewed by the applicant. In general, you should not request a letter of recommendation from someone whom you do not feel would write favorably of you, or to whom you must retell your name, but on the other hand, most people who agree to write a letter for you would only do so if they had something positive to say. If your undergraduate institution has a premedical committee, the letters usually come from this committee. Of the three letters which are typically requested, many schools prefer that two come from science faculty.

The Interview

After you have submitted complete applications, you can take a little break. Your job is almost done. Your applications are now being reviewed by the admissions committees, and if they like what they see, you will receive an invitation to interview. Congratulations—you are almost there!

*We have devoted an entire section of this book, Part Four, to the interview process.

A Note About Fees

The cost of applying to medical school can be exorbitant. Between the MCAT, the AMCAS, and the supplemental application (which averaged 13 per applicant in 2007), applying to the first school will cost a minimum of $420.

The AAMC has developed a Fee Assistance Program (FAP) to ease the financial burden for those who qualify. Note that all applicants must submit parental financial information. Applicants who were approved for assistance in 2008 received the following assistance:

- Reduction of the MCAT registration fee from $210 to $85.

- Waiver of the application fee of $520 for submitting the completed AMCAS application to up to 13 medical schools. Applicants only pay $30 for each school beyond the first 13.

In addition, most AMCAS-participating medical schools waive their supplemental application fees for applicants who have been approved for FAP.

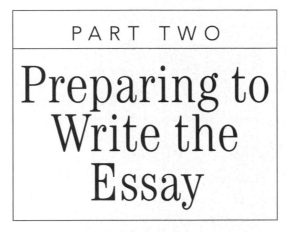

PART TWO

Preparing to Write the Essay

You have spent a lifetime becoming who you are, and now you are being asked to encapsulate the entire experience into fewer words than are generally allotted for movie reviews in your local newspaper. These few words are supposed to present your goals, motivations, sincerity, experience, and background, and do so in a concise, organized manner that accurately expresses your unique, interesting, and likeable personality. A daunting task—and yet one that every student applying to medical school is expected to do.

If you are like most people, you will approach this task in one of two ways—either you will spend weeks thinking about it, telling yourself "When I get it right in my head, then I'll write it down," or you will not think about it at all until the deadline approaches, at which point you will take a deep breath, write frantically, and hastily send it off. If you have resorted to either of these methods in the past, then you know that they are risky at best—and risk is not an element you want to introduce to a process that could dramatically change your life.

What makes both of these approaches ineffective and inefficient is that they disregard the essential first steps to writing an effective essay: planning and preparation.

The worst writing ever set down was under the influence of inspiration. Success is usually built on the completion of small incremental steps. Ask any successful writers and they will tell you, "This is hard work."

This section is designed to walk you through the steps you need before you begin writing. We offer a commonsense, step-by-step program to get you past the prewriting roadblocks of procrastination, writer's block, and sheer panic.

PART TWO

Preparing to
Write the
Essay

Assess Your Audience

Highlights

- Admissions committees are usually composed of full-time staff, faculty, students, and/or doctors from the community.
- Decisions on applicants are usually made by voting.
- Some committee members read up to 40 essays in a single day.
- Essays must be interesting, and make the committee want to interview you.
- Essays should provide proof of an applicant's motivation to become a doctor.
- Strong writing and communication skills should be demonstrated.
- Evidence of skills not found elsewhere in the application should be showcased.

<u>Do's</u>	<u>Don'ts</u>
• Make it personal	• Use gimmicks
• Use details	• Be vague
• Be honest	• Make unsubstantiated statements
• Tell stories	• Make lists
• Get feedback	• Make grammatical errors or typos

Every time you give out information, whether consciously or not, you assess your audience and you modify your delivery based on that audience. Are you writing for strangers, acquaintances, or friends? If they are strangers, what will they know about you beforehand? What are their interests and biases? What are their expectations? If these questions aren't answered for you before you begin preparation, you will have considerable difficulty deciding what to say, let alone the way in which to say it. After all, you would not address a Girl Scout troop in the same way as the U.S. Supreme Court. Now apply the same approach to your personal statement.

In this chapter we pose the questions that you should be asking about your audience, to your audience. In other words, we went out into the field and asked a variety of admissions staff at some of the top medical schools in the United States for the answers to such questions as: Who are you? What do you look for in an essay? and What are you tired of finding?

By the end of this chapter you should be familiar with the major do's and don'ts of writing an essay as defined by the very people who will later be reading and judging your essay. Think of these tips as guides to help you navigate through a vast array of options on theme, strategy, and presentation.

Knowing Your Audience

Medical school admissions committees comprise anywhere from a handful to two dozen members, and are generally made up of a combination of full-time admissions staff, faculty, students, and doctors from the community. There are often a variety of medical backgrounds represented, from clinical to general science, and from M.D.s to Ph.D.s to students. Because decisions are made by voting, this variety helps to eliminate bias and ensures that your application gets a fair trial.

Although there are a few schools that will set a cut-off point based on MCAT scores and GPA, it is rare that your application would be summarily rejected based on numbers alone. More likely, it will be read in its entirety by at least one of the members of the committee (usually one of the faculty members or second-year medical students). They will consider all aspects of your application, and if they like what they see, you will be invited to interview.

When we asked admissions officers how much time they usually spend looking at each essay during this first read, the answers ranged from three to ten minutes.

> *The time spent reading an essay can vary from a quick overview to a lengthy dissection of content and grammar. We will always look to the essay to prove interest in and research of the intended profession. If an applicant has an unexplained period of below-average grades in an otherwise strong academic record, we will look to the essay to explain the circumstances. If an applicant did some or all of their prerequisite coursework in another country, we will look to the essay to ensure strong English language skills. The standard of evaluation varies with each individual application package.*

We then asked how many statements admissions officers read in a day and their answers were surprising: Admissions officers can (and often do) churn through

40 to 50 essays a day during peak weeks. This is more than just interesting; this is important. It means that your personal statement must stand apart from dozens of others read in the same day. The same two pages that will take you days or even weeks to put together may get only a few minutes in front of the committee.

So, although we hate to say it, your personal statement needs to function both as an essay and as an advertisement. If you are not convinced, then ask yourself this: When was the last time you read over a dozen short stories in a day, spending only a few minutes on each one? Now ask: When was the last time you spent a few minutes each on a dozen or more commercials in a day? However, please do not interpret this to mean that your statement should be gimmicky, cutesy, or include a sing-a-long song.

> *When pushed, I have read 40 statements in a day. That means that by the end of the day, I've developed a very low tolerance to nonsense.*

What it does mean is that the best essays, like the best ads, are going to be interesting enough to grab the reader's attention on the first read and powerful enough to hold it even if it's the fortieth essay the reader has read that day. But unlike an ad, the essay must also withstand longer, more in-depth scrutiny.

What the Admissions Committee Is Looking For

During that first, quick look at your file (transcripts, science and nonscience GPAs, MCAT scores, application, recommendations, and personal statement), what the admissions committee seeks is essentially the same:

1. Proven ability to succeed.
2. Clear intellectual ability, analytical and critical thinking skills.
3. Evidence that this person has the potential to make not only a good medical student, but a good doctor.

But the committee is looking for more than this in the essay specifically. We will discuss in detail the essay issues that were unanimously listed as most important by our admissions committee.

Motivation

Your application to medical school is a testimony to your desire to ultimately be a doctor. The admissions committee will look at your essay to see that you've answered the obvious, but not so simple, question "Why?" You must be able to explain your *motivation* for attending medical school.

I look for a sustained understanding of why the candidate wants to enter medicine, how they've tested their interest, and how they've prepared for medical school.

Touch on your passion to pursue medicine. For many, medicine is akin to a calling, and the evaluator must get a sense that they are hearing and responding to the same motivation.

You will be offered much advice in the upcoming pages, with plenty of do's and don'ts. In the midst of all this, whatever you do, do not lose sight of the ultimate goal of the essay—to convince the admissions committee members that you belong at their medical school. Everything we tell you should be used as a means to this end, so step back from the details of this process regularly and remind yourself of the big picture:

The essay is the way for candidates to make the argument as to why they, among all the highly qualified candidates, should be admitted to medical school and the eventual practice of medicine.

Writing/Communication Skills

Another obvious function of the essay is to showcase your *language abilities* and *writing skills.*

In the essay I want a clear sense that they understand and can communicate well why they are compelling candidates.

Especially if an applicant did some or all of the prerequisite coursework in another country, we will look to the essay to ensure strong English language skills.

At this level, good writing skills are not sought; they are expected. So, while a beautifully written essay alone isn't going to get you into medical school, a poorly written one could keep you out.

Beyond showcasing your writing abilities and demonstrating your motivation, what else can the essay do for you? Following is more of what the members of the committee hope to find when they read your essay.

Soft Skills

Let the rest of your application, not the personal statement, speak for your *hard* skills and achievements (such as your academic excellence, your fantastic MCAT scores, your class rank). What admissions officers seek in the essay are some specific *soft* skills such as sincerity, maturity, empathy, compassion, and motivation. These qualities were rated especially high in the medical community, more so than for any other graduate-level program we studied.

YOUR SOFTER SIDE: PERSONAL QUALITIES SOUGHT BY MEDICAL ADMISSIONS STAFF		
(Listed according to the number of times the qualities were mentioned)		
1.	2.	3.
motivation	diversity	sensitivity
commitment	uniqueness	communication skills
sincerity	interest	humanitarian beliefs
honesty	compassion	enthusiasm
maturity	empathy	creativity

Because these qualities are not quantifiable, and therefore not easily demonstrated through the usual criteria of grades and numbers, the essay is your first opportunity (and one of your only ones) to showcase them.

All of the essays we have included demonstrate in one way or another that the writers have the soft skills necessary to be good doctors. A few of them even come right out and say it, as in Essay 31:

> *Motivation, independence, maturity, precisely those qualities my experiences in Eastern Europe instilled, will be essential to a fruitful career.*

When qualities are mentioned as directly as this, the applicant must be careful to support the claims with clear evidence gathered from personal experience. More often, applicants let their achievements and experiences speak for themselves, and the qualities that they demonstrate are inferred. Essay 8, for example, never directly touts humanism, maturity, or sincerity. But after reading about his intimate and enduring involvement in the lives of three boys through his volunteer experiences, you would not doubt that the writer is in strong possession of all three.

A Real Person

This list is not ordered by importance; if it were, this category would be listed first. What our admissions officers said they seek more than any specific skill or characterisic mentioned in the personal statement is a real, live human being:

> *The members of a medical admissions committee are responsible for choosing the next generation of medical doctors. These are the people who will be healing our children, curing us and our parents, and literally saving lives. Put it in that perspective and the responsibility we feel is enormous. For this reason, we're going to choose to accept someone we feel we know, trust, and like.*

In light of this, then, it might not surprise you that when we asked admissions officers and medical students for their number one piece of advice regarding the essay, we received the same response almost every time. Although it was expressed in many different ways (be honest, be sincere, be unique, be personal, and so on) it all came down to the same point: "Be Yourself!"

> *My number one piece of advice is: Be yourself when you write the essay. The medical profession is a lifetime commitment. Let those in the profession know what drives you towards it!*

Unfortunately, achieving this level of communication in writing does not come naturally to everyone, but that does not mean it cannot be learned. Part of what can make this kind of writing seem so difficult is that it is very hard to gauge the impressions you are creating through your writing. Even if you have followed every tip in this book, it is a good idea to have some objective people—preferably those who do not already know you well—read it over when you have finished. Ask them if they got a sense of the kind of person you are, or if they were able to picture you as they were reading. How accurate is their description relative to the one you were trying to present? Then ask them if the essay conveyed the type of person they would trust in a life or death situation.

Get Personal

The only way to let the admissions committee see you as an individual is to make your essay personal. When you do this, your essay will automatically be more interesting and engaging, helping it stand out from the hundreds of others the committee will be reviewing that week.

> *After reading hundreds of essays in my time on the Harvard Medical School admissions committee, I would tell people a couple of key things. First, make it personal. The most boring, dry essays are those that go on about how the applicant loves science and working with people and wants to serve humanity, but offer few personal details that give a sense of what the applicant is like.*

> *Personalize your essay as much as possible—generic essays are not only boring to read, they're a waste of time because they don't tell you anything about the applicant that helps you get to know them better.*

What does it mean to make your essay personal? It means that you drop the formalities and write about something that is truly meaningful to you. It means that you include a story or anecdote taken from your life, using ample detail and colorful imagery to give it life. And it means, above all, being completely honest.

This book contains many examples of essays that get personal, including Essay 33. The writer begins by recollecting her experience with anorexia and her admiration for the doctor who saved her life. But it is more than the story that makes her essay real—it is the way that she describes her experiences. She uses a personal tone throughout the essay, for example when she describes herself while volunteering at an AIDS clinic:

> *. . . I am constantly reminded of how much I have to learn. I look at a baby and notice its cute, pudgy toes. Dr. V. plays with it while conversing with its mother, and in less than a minute has noted its responsiveness, strength, and attachment to its parent, and checked its reflexes, color and hydration. Gingerly, I search for the tympanic membrane in the ears of a cooperative child and touch an infant's warm, soft belly, willing my hands to have a measure of Dr. V.'s competence.*

It is her admittance that she doesn't yet know everything she needs to know coupled with the picture she paints of herself noticing a baby's "cute pudgy toes" and "gingerly" searching in "the ears of a cooperative child" and touching "an infant's warm, soft belly." As readers, we do not have to strain to create a mental image of the author as a caring, still somewhat tentative individual. This vivid portrayal is painted by a series of personal details.

Just as this writer did not rely on her story of anorexia to make her essay personal, one admissions officer comments:

> *A personal epiphany, tragedy, life change, or earth-shattering event is not essential to a strong essay.*

This point cannot be stressed enough. Personal does not necessarily mean heavy, or emotional, or awe inspiring. It is a small minority of students who will truly have had a life-changing event to write about. Perhaps they have spent time living abroad or have experienced death or disease from close proximity. But this is the exception and not the rule.

In fact, students who rely too heavily on these weighty experiences often do themselves an injustice. They often don't think about what has really touched them or interests them because they are preoccupied with the topic that they think will impress the committee. They write about their grandfather's death because they think that only death (or the emotional equivalent) is significant enough to make them seem introspective and mature. What often happens, however, is that they rely on the experience itself to speak for them and never explain what it meant to them or give a solid example of how it was emotionally influencing. In other words, they don't make it personal.

Details, Details, Details

To make your essay personal, learn from the example above and *use details*. Show, don't tell, who you are by backing your claims with real experiences.

> *Essays only really help you if they are unique and enable the reader to get a sense of who you are based on examples and scenarios and ideas, rather than lists of what you've done. The readers want to find out who this person is, not what the person has done, although the two are obviously interrelated.*

The key words from this quote are *examples, scenarios,* and *ideas*. Using detail means being specific. Each and every point that you make needs to be backed up by specific instances taken from your experience. It is these details that make your story unique and interesting. Although it is true that the use of excessive detail can bog down the pace of a story, don't even think about limiting the amount that you incorporate during the first phases of writing. Too much detail in your writing is a much less likely pitfall than the alternative. To begin, err on the side of too much information and you can trim it down later. This way you won't find yourself manufacturing details to fit neatly into an essay you thought was complete, but that turned out to be less than engaging.

Look at the detail used by the writer of Essay 23, for example. She describes herself gently rocking her first patient, "taking care not to disturb the jumbled array of tubes that overwhelmed his tiny body," and says that she has "worked with everything from papier mache to popsicle sticks" and that the children in her ward talk about "Nintendo or the latest Disney movie." These details create a personal, interesting story out of what might have been a yawn-inducing account that could be attributed to any of a thousand applicants.

Tell a Story

Tell a story. It always makes for more interesting reading and it usually conveys something more personal than such blanket statements as "I want to help people."

Incorporating a story into your essay can be a great way to make it interesting and enjoyable. The safest and most common way of integrating a story into an essay is to *tell the story* first, then step back into the role of narrator and explain why it was presented and what lessons were learned. The reason this method works is that it forces you to begin with the action, which is a sure way to get the readers' attention and keep them reading.

Many of the essay examples in this book make effective use of storytelling. Essay 17 begins with a storm at sea, Essay 7 begins with a tale of stage fright before a theater performance, and Essay 13 begins with a newspaper clipping about the writer as a child. The writer of Essay 30 takes an even more creative approach to the story method by incorporating the tale of a prehistoric woman whose bones he has analyzed. What all these writers understood is that a story is best used to draw the reader in, and it should always relate back to the motivation to attend medical school or the ability to succeed once admitted.

Be Honest!

This last point comes with no caveats, and should be upheld without exception. Nothing could be more simple, more straightforward, or more crucial than this: *Be honest,* forthright, and sincere.

If you say that one of your favorite hobbies is playing chess, then you better have a favorite opening move; your interviewer might be an expert player and want to swap techniques!

Admissions officers have zero tolerance for hype. If you try to be something that you're not, it will be apparent to the committee. You will give the impression of being immature at best and unethical at worst.

I served on the Harvard Medical School admissions committee, and can say that it is very important to be honest. The students will be asked many times about the personal statement when interviewing, and it's painfully obvious when they exaggerate or are overly dramatic when recounting their experiences.

When you are honest about your motivations and goals, you will come across as more personable and real. Essay 21, for example, begins:

When I entered Dartmouth College in 1987, I was amazed by the large number of students already labeled as "premeds." I wondered how those students were able to decide with such certainty that they wanted to study medicine, and I imagined that they all must have known from a very early age that they would one day be great doctors. I had no such inklings, and if asked as a child what I wanted to be when I grew up, I would have said that I wanted to be an Olympic skier or soccer player.

Because of the numerous essays that begin: "I've wanted to be a doctor for as long as I can remember. . ." this writer's honest approach was refreshing and memorable.

What the Admissions Committee Is Tired of Reading

Not surprisingly, much of what admissions officers are tired of finding is simply the converse of what they hope to receive. In other words: Don't be generic, don't lie, and don't hand in a poorly written, ill-constructed document riddled with grammatical errors.

There were, however, a few pet peeves that were cited so frequently by admissions officers that they bear repeating. After all, they wouldn't be pet peeves if people weren't still doing them.

Gimmicks

When it comes to creativity, the consensus among our admissions team was clear: Interesting is good; gimmicky is bad. To put it plainly, don't give in to *gimmicks*. The problem is in knowing where to draw the line. According to one admissions officer, "What might have been cute at the college level of admissions simply won't cut it at this level of competition." To complicate matters more is the inevitability that admissions officers will disagree among themselves about where to draw the line.

Here are two attention-getters that definitely flopped:

One applicant used a computer program to craft her essay in the form of a tooth, with roots and all. What a mess! You couldn't even figure out how one line followed another.

You could write a whole book on the gimmicks alone. The student who mailed via UPS an actual front door with a sneaker glued to it, painted with the words "I just want to get my foot in the door" might better have spent his creative energies figuring out how to raise his 1.8 GPA.

Contrast the above with one example of a person who did it right:

One essay that caught my eye began "I was raised by Donald Duck." I was intrigued and went on to read this excellent essay that explained how the applicant's father used his Donald Duck voice to soothe the fears of the children who were his patients, and how this personal touch influenced the son to pursue the same career. He then tied it together nicely by ending up with ". . .and I could do worse than grow up to be Donald Duck." This essay showed the applicant to be well researched in the field, intelligent, and creative.

If you are considering taking a creative approach, consider that maturity is valued higher than any of the following qualities by admissions committees: creativity, interest, innovation, or initiative. So, when in doubt, err on the conservative side.

One example of an applicant who took a risk (if only a slight one) is in Essay 4. The writer begins by using quotes of people describing why they fell in love, and then uses them to draw a metaphor between medical school and marriage. She risks sounding trite, but she is able to pull it off by moving briskly from the metaphor into solid demonstrations of her motivation, her achievements, and her experience. She also brings the last line back to the original metaphor, which both justifies its use and makes for a satisfying read.

Mechanical Errors

There is absolutely no excuse for mechanical errors such as poor grammar or misspellings. One unforgivable error is the mistake of forgetting to replace the proper name of the school throughout the statement. Harvard consistently gets essays beginning, "The reason I want to attend Stanford. . ."

Here is some of the advice given by admissions staff and students alike:

Proofread! Have others proofread! Spell check! It's stunning how many people have careless, even really obvious typos in their statements. It makes the applicant look sloppy, uninterested, unintelligent.

Don't cram your essay onto the page with a tiny font. If I can't read it without a magnifying glass, I won't read it at all.

Stay away from lots of SAT-type big vocabulary words. It's obvious which applicants wrote their essays with the thesaurus in hand.

Actually answer the question asked. Many people just list off their accomplishments and never relate it to the theme of the question.

Get Feedback

This has been mentioned several times already but it bears repeating: It is imperative that you get feedback about your essays before submitting your final version. For a variety of reasons, many of the don'ts listed above are hard to spot in your own writing. Find an honest, objective person to read the entire essay set for each school. As comforting as it might be, do not accept "It's great!" as feedback. Ask the reader to look specifically for the do's and don'ts listed in this chapter and to recount to you the main points you were trying to make. Have the reader describe his or her impression of your strengths and weaknesses. Approach the reader a week after he or she has read the essays and see what (if anything) has remained memorable. Finally, if your proofreaders are not familiar with what a successful admissions essay looks like, have them read some of the examples from this book in order to have a measuring stick by which to judge your work.

Finally, do not rely on only one person's opinion, especially if you know the person well or disagree with the points the person may have made. Even the most objective readers have their own set of biases and opinions, and no one person can accurately predict the reception your writing will have at the school to which you are applying.

One way to offset this potential risk is to make one of your evaluations a professional one. Keep in mind that almost everyone gets feedback on their essays. Seeking that help from professionals assures that the advice you are getting on essay content is based on evidence of what admissions committees are looking for and that grammatical feedback is coming from people with solid editorial experience. The authors of this book, with help from admissions officers and experienced editors, created a website for this purpose. At *Ivyessays.com*, you can upload your essay and choose different levels of feedback depending on where you are in the writing process. If you are only in the rough draft phase of putting your thoughts together, you can submit your essay for "quick feedback." You don't need to worry about the grammar or mechanics at this stage. Editors will focus on the content of your essay and will send you tips and advice on how to improve it. If you are further along in the process, you can submit the essay for a "full edit" and editors will help you polish your essay to perfection.

Gather Your Material

Highlights
- Read through essays that have been proven to work (included in this book).
- Use brainstorming exercises in this section to help devise essay topics.
- Assess yourself by writing down experiences, accomplishments, and skills.
- Make notes of your major influences.
- Clearly identify your goals.
- Scan your notes for the topics that best describe you and your motivations.
- Identify the topics that would make the most interesting essay.

Now that you have a better understanding of your readers and some of their opinions about what makes an essay exceptionally good or bad, you may feel ready to begin writing. You may even feel inspired about a particular topic and have some good ideas for presenting it. But before you begin typing, stop for a moment and assess your situation.

Creating an essay full of imagery and detail will require you to think carefully about your subject matter before you begin to write. This means much more than simply knowing the points you want to make. It means, first and foremost, that you know yourself. Interesting, reflective, and revealing essays are always the result of careful self-analysis. Second, it means that you understand the specific points you wish to make in your essay and have identified concrete details to use in support of each of these points. We often forget the details of our lives over time, yet it is these details that will provide the material for your essay, making it vibrant and alive.

This chapter contains a number of brainstorming activities designed to help you get to know yourself better and gather the material you will need to write a colorful essay. The first step in this process can actually be a fun one. Sit back and read through examples of essays that have gotten previous applicants into medical school. It is not only informative, allowing you to size up the competition; the experiences that other applicants have written about may spark memories that you had not considered writing about before. After you've had your fill of what has worked for others, we are going to ask you to begin a series of creative writing exercises. The exercises in this section will offer solutions to open the channels of your mind and get your pen moving. If you are not having a problem getting started, you might want to skip this section and go straight to "Assess Yourself."

Seek Inspiration Through Examples

We believe that it can be enormously helpful at this stage of the process, to peruse examples of essays that have already been proven to work. We have compiled more than 35 essays that applicants have actually submitted in their medical school application packages; each of these applicants has been accepted. We have not made any changes to these essays. We don't claim that they are perfect, but we can at least claim that they were effective. By reading through any number of these essays you may find inspiration to write your own essays. Many different themes are included and different levels of writing skills are represented. You may even use this opportunity to pretend that you are on an admissions committee, reading through multiple essays in a day. Which ones bore you and which ones make you want to meet the author? Take a clue from the good ones and try to develop a similar style. Through creative and effective writing, almost any subject can be made interesting—just remember to be honest and to draw from your own experiences.

Creative Writing Exercises

To get the most benefit out of this section, put your anxieties aside. Do not think about what the admissions committee wants, or worry about grammar or style—and especially do not worry about what anyone would think. These worries hamper spontaneity and creativity, and besides, no one ever has to see these exercises anyway. Focus instead on writing quickly and recording every thought you have the instant you have it. You will know that you are performing these exercises correctly if you are relaxing and having fun.

The Inventory

This exercise is designed to get your pen moving. The goal is simply to compile an inventory of your activities and accomplishments—school, sports, extracurricular activities, awards, work, and pastimes. You may have already made a similar list during the application process. If so, start with that list and try to add to it. This list will become fodder for topics to use when writing your personal statement. During this exercise you do not need to write down any qualities, skills, or feelings associated with the activities. For now it is more important to be completely comprehensive in the breadth of topics and items you include. For example, if you taught yourself chess or particularly enjoy occasional chess games with your uncle, you do not need to be in a chess club or have won a trophy to add it to the list. Think of how you spend your time each and every day, and include any items that seem significant to you. Spend no less than twenty minutes writing, and keep going for up to an hour if you can. If you run out of items quickly, don't worry—you will probably come up with more during the other exercises.

Stream of Consciousness

Take twenty minutes to answer each of the questions: Who are you? and What do you want? Start with whatever comes to mind first, and write without pausing for the entire time. Do not limit yourself to any one area of your life such as your career. Just let yourself go, be honest, and have fun. You might be surprised by what kind of results can come from this type of free association.

Morning Pages

Keep paper and a pen at your bedside. Set your alarm clock twenty minutes early, and when you are still in bed and groggy with sleep, start writing. Write about anything that comes to mind, as fast as you can, and do not stop until you have filled a page or two.

Journal Writing

Keep a journal, especially if you are stuck and your brainstorming seems to be going nowhere. Record not what you do each day, but your responses and thoughts to each day's experiences. You may learn more about yourself through everyday experiences and your feelings about them than you would imagine.

Top Tens

Write down your top ten favorites in the following areas: movies, books, plays, sports, paintings, historical eras, famous people. Step back and look at the lists objectively. What do they say about you? Do you see a pattern, or do any particular passions present themselves? And finally, have any of your favorites had a significant effect on your outlook, opinions, or direction?

Free-Flow Writing

Choose one word that seems to appear on many of your questions such as *influence, strengths, career, diversity,* or *goals,* and brainstorm around that word. Set a timer for ten minutes and write without stopping. Write down everything you can think of that relates to the topic, including any single words that come to mind.

Assess Yourself

If the exercises in the last section have successfully stirred your thoughts and animated your pen, then it is time to impose more focus on your brainstorming. These next exercises help you do just that. They are more concentrated on finding the specific points and details that you will need to incorporate into your statement. But be sure to retain the open mind and creative attitude fostered in the last section.

The Chronological Method

Start from childhood and record any and all special or pivotal experiences that you remember. Go from grade to grade, and job to job, noting any significant lessons learned, achievements reached, painful moments endured, or obstacles overcome. Also, include your feelings about those occurrences as you remember them. If you are a visual person, it might help to draw a timeline. Do not leave out any significant event.

The goal of this exercise is to help you uncover long-forgotten material from your youth. This material can be used to demonstrate a long-standing dedication to the medical field, or to illustrate the kind of person you are by painting an image of yourself as a child. Be cautioned in advance, though, that relying too heavily on accomplishments or awards from too far in your past can diminish the strength of your points. Medical schools are more interested in what you have been doing since college than in what you accomplished, no matter how impressive, in high school.

Assess Your Accomplishments

Write down anything you are proud of doing, no matter how small or insignificant it might seem. Do not limit your achievements to your career. If you have overcome a difficult personal obstacle, be sure to list this too. If something is important to you, it speaks volumes about who you are and what makes you tick. Some accomplishments will be obvious, such as any achievement that received public accolade or acknowledgment. Others are less so, and many times the most defining moments of our lives are those we are inclined to dismiss.

List Your Skills

Do an assessment of your skills that is similar to the one you did for your accomplishments. Do not limit yourself to your "medical" skills such as helping people or research abilities. Cast your net broadly. Being able to draw connections between your unique skills and how they will make you a good doctor is what will make you memorable. Think about the MCAT during this exercise. This test is designed to gauge certain quantifiable skills. Think of other skills that are not specifically tested, such as professionalism, and emphasize strengths in these areas. Begin by looking back at the last exercise and listing the skills that are highlighted by your accomplishments. When you have a list of words, start brainstorming on other ways you have demonstrated these skills in the last few years. Pretend that you are defending these skills in front of a panel of judges. Stop only when you have proven each point to the best of your ability.

Analyze Personality Traits

There is a fine and fuzzy line between skills and personality traits that can be used to your advantage. Almost any quality can be positioned as a skill or ability if the right examples are used to demonstrate them. If you had trouble listing and defending your skills in the last exercise, then shift the focus to your qualities and characteristics instead. Make a few columns on a sheet of paper. In the first one, list some adjectives you would use to describe yourself. In the next one, list the words your best friend would use. Use the other columns for other types of people—perhaps one for your boss and another for family members or coworkers.

When you have finished, see which words come up the most often. Look for such words as maturity, responsibility, sense of purpose, academic ability, intellectual curiosity, creativity, thoughtfulness, trustworthiness, sense of humor, perseverance, commitment, integrity, enthusiasm, confidence, conscientiousness, candor, leadership, goal-orientation, independence, and tact, to name a few. Group them together and list the different situations in which you have exhibited these characteristics. How effectively can you illustrate or prove that you possess these qualities? How do these qualities reflect on your ability to succeed in the medical world?

Note Major Influences

You can refer back to your Top Ten lists for help getting started with this exercise. Was there a particular person who shaped your values and views? Did a particular book or quote make you rethink your life? Relationships can be good material for an essay, particularly a relationship that challenged you to look at people in a different way. Perhaps you had a wise and generous mentor from whom you learned a great deal. Have you had an experience that changed how you see the world, or defines who you are? What details of your life, special achievements, and pivotal events have helped shape you and influence your goals?

Identify Your Goals

The first step of this exercise is to let loose and write down anything that comes to mind regarding your goals: What are your dreams? What did you want to be when you were younger? If you could do or be anything right now, regardless of skill, money, or other restrictions, what would it be? Think as broadly as you wish, and do not limit yourself to professional goals. Will you have kids? Will you travel? Where would you like to live?

The second step is to begin honing in on some more specific or realistic goals. Given your current skills, education, and experience, where could you expect to be in twenty years? Where would you be ideally? Think in terms of five-year increments, listing actual positions and places, if possible. Be detailed and thorough in your assessment, and when you think you are finished, dig a little deeper.

Your goal of becoming a doctor is obvious, of course, but when you can show the admissions committee that you have thought more specifically about your goals, it reemphasizes the sincerity of your motivation. It also reassures the committee that you understand what becoming a doctor means specifically, that it is more than being a hero and getting to write M.D. after your name.

At this and every stage of brainstorming, do not hesitate to expand and modify lists that you created previously. If at this stage of the process you realize that a strong influence in your life was not in your original list, that doesn't mean it is any less important to you. Add it now. The subconscious mind has an interesting way of retrieving information like this, and the brainstorming process is meant to uncover as much of it as possible, in whatever way it surfaces.

Before You Move On . . .

Knowing yourself and all of your goals thoroughly can be difficult. Not all of your motivations, significant influences, defining experiences, or career goals—especially long-term—are going to be completely clear to you at this point. However, if these exercises proved more than a little difficult for you, it could be a sign that you need to step back and reassess your decision to seek an M.D. Because expressing your reasons for applying to medical school is so central to the medical essay, giving vague motivations will indicate ambivalence to the committee, and that alone could ruin your chances of getting into medical school.

On the other hand, if this chapter was successful for you, you should now have plenty of material—in fact, more than you need—to write successful and convincing essays. The next chapter, "Develop a Strategy," will help you understand how to present this material as a cohesive whole, leaving the committee with a strong sense of who you are and a persuasive, targeted argument for why it should accept you.

Develop a Strategy

Highlights

- A strong personal statement will include why you want to be a doctor, how you are unique, and details of your qualifications and experiences.
- Multiple themes should be woven into a cohesive and well-structured essay.
- All themes related to motivations and qualifications should be evidenced by experiences and achievements, not words alone.

<u>Do's</u>

- Do explain a particular weakness in your application if you have a strong justification.
- Do showcase unique talents that may be outside the medical field.

<u>Don'ts</u>

- Don't let excuses for weaknesses be the primary theme of your essay.
- Don't turn your essay into a prose form of your "curriculum vitae (C.V.)."

At this stage you should have plenty of material from which to build your personal statement. This means that you have a solid understanding of your objectives—both personal and professional—and your motivations for going to medical school, and that you have plenty of details to back them up. The details should comprise specific examples from your past—the summer spent researching tribal cultures in the Amazon, your volunteer experience as a literacy tutor, the time you were ten and healed the wing of an injured pigeon.

Now it is time to mesh these disparate details of your life into a cohesive whole. This chapter represents the final stage of preparation, and the last step you need to take before you begin to write the first draft of your essay. In it, you will identify your themes and develop your strategy.

Identify Your Themes

Part of what makes the personal statement so difficult is that you need to do so much in one essay. Unlike the college application essay, where your motivation is unquestioned and your goals can remain undefined, and unlike other graduate programs where you are expected to write multiple essays in response to specific questions, writing a personal statement requires that you incorporate multiple themes in one composition. Needless to say, this can be tricky.

There are three basic themes that need to be incorporated into your essay:

1. Why you want to be a doctor

2. What makes you unique or exceptional

3. What your qualifications and experiences are

In addition, if you received poor grades in some of your required coursework but otherwise have a strong application, admissions committees expect this to be explained in the essay. If you have no explanation, you may not wish to attempt it but if there were extenuating circumstances, you should strive to incorporate this topic into your essay. It should not be an actual theme, because, as such, your essay would probably not be very uplifting or interesting. However, it should at least be mentioned in one paragraph and tied as seamlessly as possible to the other essay themes.

There are several different ways to approach each of the themes mentioned above. The more common of these approaches are outlined below with tips and advice for how to best handle each approach.

Theme 1: Why You Want to Be a Doctor

Many people look back in time to find the moment of their initial inspiration. Some people have wanted to be a doctor for so long they do not even know what originally inspired them. To incorporate this theme, look back to the material you gathered in the last chapter, specifically in response to "The Chronological Method," "Note Major Influences," and "Identify Your Goals." Ask yourself these questions: How old was I when I first wanted to become a doctor? Was there a defining moment? Was there ever any ambivalence? Was I inspired by a specific person? What kind of doctor do I want to be and how does that tie into my motivation?

Here are a few of the common ways that students incorporate this theme:

"I've Always Wanted to Be a Doctor"

AKA: "I've Wanted to Be a Doctor Since I Was. . ." and "Everyone Has Always Said I'd Be a Doctor"

This is perhaps the most common approach of all. The secret to doing it well is to show, not just tell, why you want to be a doctor. You cannot just say it and expect it to stand on its own.

The "I've always wanted to be a doctor" essay has been done to death. I think candidates need to be careful to show that their decision was not only a preadolescent one and has been tested over the years and approached in a mature manner.

Supply believable details from your life to make your desire real to the reader. One secret to avoiding the "here we go again" reaction is to be particularly careful with your first line. Starting with "I've wanted to be a doctor since. . ." makes the reader cringe. It's an easy line to fall back on, but admissions officers have read this sentence more times than they care to count; don't become another statistic.

See Essays 5, 13, 29, and 35 for some examples of successfully incorporating this theme. All of the writers use solid examples to back themselves up, and none of them depend on this theme alone to carry the essay.

"My Parents Are Doctors"

This approach to the "why I want to be a doctor" theme is dangerous for a different reason.

It's a prejudice of mine, but the legacy essay, the one that reads, "My dad and my grandpa and my great-grandpa were all doctors so I should be too," makes me suspect immaturity. I envision young people who can't think for themselves or make up their own minds.

This is not the opinion of every officer, though. The point is not to avoid admitting that your parent is an M.D., it is to avoid depending on that as the sole reason for you wanting to go to medical school. If a parent truly was your inspiration, then describe exactly why you were inspired. Essay 33 tells of inspiration from a mentor: The doctor in this case is not related to her, but the treatment is still applicable.

Essayists 12, 22, 24, 27, and 35 also discuss a physician in the family but none dwells on it and most only mention it circumstantially. Essay 22 has a unique approach; the writer tells of how he initially revolted against becoming a doctor because of family pressure to do so. His story of how he eventually came around to the decision on his own terms makes for an interesting and convincing read.

"My Doctor Changed My Life!"

AKA: "Being a Patient Made Me Want to Become a Doctor"

Some people claim to be motivated to become doctors because they have had personal experience of illness or disability.

I had a student who grew up with a chronic illness. She spent much time with physicians and other health care providers throughout her young life. In her essay she wrote about this continuing experience and how the medical professionals treated her. She wrote of her admiration of them as well as her understanding that they couldn't yet cure her. Her essay literally jumped off the page as being unique to her and a compelling understanding of and testament to her desire to join the people who had been so important to her life.

If your personal experience with the medical profession sincerely is your motivation for attending medical school, then do write about it. The problem is that many students fall back on this topic even when it does not particularly hold true for them. We cannot stress enough that you do not have to have a life-defining experience to have an exciting statement. Admissions committees receive piles of accident and illness-related essays and the ones that seem insincere stick out like sore thumbs (pun intended!) and do not reflect well on you as a candidate.

"My endocrinologist changed my life!" "My dermatologist gave me my confidence back!" These types of themes are certainly valid, but go beyond that to what particular aspect of the profession intrigues you. Do you understand how many years of study your endocrinologist had to have in order to reach his level of practice? Have you observed your dermatologist for any significant amount of time? Do you know that the profession now is much different than it was when he or she was starting out? Have you given any thought to the danger of infectious diseases to all health-care professionals? Present a well-organized, complete essay dealing with these points.

Essayists 9, 15, 18, and 33 all found motivation, in varying degrees, for becoming doctors when they were being treated themselves. The writer of Essay 9 mentions his experience only briefly toward the end of his essay. He uses it as a confirmation of his decision to be a doctor (instead of as his primary motivation) and demonstrates that because of the experience he will become a better doctor.

Essayist 15 uses the theme less subtly, but it works nicely. He begins with a line that is often overused, and makes it the subject of the first paragraph:

Ironically, the first time I seriously considered becoming a doctor was as a patient.

What makes it work is that he moves briskly in the next paragraph toward demonstrating that he balanced his initial inspiration with real hospital experience. This taught him that being a physician is more about hard work and commitment than about the good feeling of being cured or curing.

Essay 18 describes the writer's experience with illness in vivid language to capture the reader's interest:

The morning of New Year's Day, 1978, was bright and sunny. Refreshed from a good night's sleep, I lifted the blankets, rose to my feet, and collapsed, unable to walk.

The writer does not dwell on the experience, though, and like the others provides plenty of further evidence of her sincere motivation.

Essay 33 demonstrates the most personal patient experience of them all: The writer suffered from anorexia and "slowly came to realize that my pediatrician had saved my life—despite my valiant efforts to the contrary." Her story works because she tells it objectively and with no intention to manipulate the reader's emotions.

"My Mom Had Cancer"

This theme is really just a variation of "I was a patient myself" and the same advice applies: If a loved one's battle with illness, trauma, or disability is truly what inspired your wish to become a doctor, then by all means mention it. But don't dwell on it, don't overdramatize, and don't let it stand as your sole motivation—show that you've done your research and you understand the life of a doctor and you chose it for a variety of reasons.

Essayists 2, 3, 16, 18, 27, 32, and 34 all have had someone close to them suffer physically in some way. They each approach the subject differently. Essayists 3 and 32, for example, both mention very briefly how a sister struggled (one with cancer and one with retardation), but neither spends more than a couple of sentences on the subject. Essayists 2 and 27 both begin with their mothers' recoveries as a way to draw the reader in, and show proof of an early motivation to heal. Essay 16 begins with the story of a teacher suffering from AIDS. What validates this focus is the writer's subsequent involvement as a volunteer at an HIV clinic. Without this evidence to prove her sincerity, the poignancy of the situation would have been doubted and the essay considerably weakened.

Pitfall Number 1: The Hard-Luck Tale

Some truly outstanding essays are about strong emotional experiences such as a childhood struggle with disease or the death of a loved one. Some of these are done so effectively that they are held up as role models for all essays.

I had a student who was considered a weak candidate because of poor grades and low test scores. She was African-American and although she had pursued all the right avenues (classes, MCAT, volunteer experiences) to prepare herself for medical school, she remained undistinguished as a candidate— until, that is, she wrote her essay. The essay revealed her tremendous and sincere drive. She was from a crime-riddled area of New York City and several of her siblings had been violently killed. She wrote about her experience and her desire to practice medicine in the city and improve the neighborhood where she was raised. It was compelling, believable, and truly inspiring.

While it is true that these poignant tales can provide very strong evidence of motivation for medical school, they are difficult to do well and need to be handled with extreme care and sensitivity. And, as we have said before, do not rely on the tale itself to carry you through; always clearly demonstrate your motivation.

This is going to sound harsh, but I don't like the tales of woe such as the ones that begin with the mother's death from cancer. Frankly, I feel manipulated and I don't think that the personal statement is the proper mode of expression for that kind of emotion.

"I Want to Help People"

It is common and natural to cite a desire to help people. Essays 8, 14, and 34 do just this. Essay 8 is perhaps the most poignant and convincing of the group. The reader is convinced of the writer's sincerity based on the depth of his involvement with three boys as part of a volunteer program. It is easy to see how such a person would make a kind, caring, and involved physician. Essayist 34 compares being a doctor to being a minister; it rings sincere when we discover that he himself is an elder in his church.

The Medical Dichotomy

One of the major draws of the medical field is its dualistic nature combining hard-core science with the softer side of helping people. This is described by people in many ways; some describe it as a dichotomy of science to art; to others it is intellectualism to humanism, theory to application, research to creativity, or qualitative to social skills. No matter how you choose to phrase it, if you mention the dichotomy, then be sure to touch on your qualifications and experience in both areas. Essayist 9 begins:

> *Medicine and technology are becoming increasingly intertwined. The field has moved from the days of simple X-rays to implantable medication dispensers and gene therapy.*

He goes on to detail his experience in aerospace and biomedical engineering as well as his time spent as a volunteer and later as an EMT in a hospital. So he doesn't just draw an analogy between the two fields, he discusses his experience in both and the fact that he wants to continue to work in a branch of medicine that utilizes technology (and how) throughout the essay. Essays 1, 4, 5, 9, 12, 15, 22, 25, and 26 all mention one or more of these contrasts and tie them into their motivation or aptitude for the study of medicine.

Theme 2: What Makes You Unique or Exceptional

This theme is often tied in closely with "why you are a qualified person." Be very clear on the difference, though; the latter focuses specifically on your experience (medical or otherwise) that qualifies you to be a better medical student, while the former focuses strictly on you as a person. Committees are always on the lookout for well-rounded candidates. They want to see that you are interesting, involved, and tied to the community around you.

To help you think about how to support this theme, look at your answers to the exercises from the last chapter and ask yourself: What makes me different? Do I have any special talents or abilities that might make me more interesting? How will my skills and personality traits add diversity to the class? What makes me stand out from the crowd? How will this help me to be a better physician and student?

If you are creative, you'll be able to take whatever makes you different—even a flaw—and turn it to your advantage.

One student wrote about her experience as a childhood "klutz" and how her many accidents kept her continually seeking medical care. The care she received was the impetus to her desire to become a doctor and made her essay entertaining, sincere, and eminently credible.

Note that the candidate in this example tied her experience to her desire to become a doctor. It is imperative that this be done with practically every point you make in your essay.

The Talented Among Us

If you are one of a lucky few who have an outstanding talent or ability, now is no time to hide it. Whether you are a star athlete, an opera singer, or a violin virtuoso, by all means make it a focus of your essay.

These people can be some of the strongest of candidates. Assuming, always, that they've excelled in the required preparatory coursework, the other strengths can take them over the top. Athletes, musicians, and others can make the compelling case of excellence, achievement, discipline, mastering a subject/talent and leveraging their abilities. Medical schools are full of these types; they thrive by bringing high achievers who possess intellectual ability into their realm.

If you do plan to focus on a strength outside the field of medicine, your challenge becomes one of how to tie the experience of that ability into your motivation for becoming a doctor.

Essays 6, 10, 11, 18, and 32 were all written by people with musical ability. Essay 6 begins with a description of an African drum performance during a Catholic Mass, and then ties nicely back to the musical theme in the last line. Music was a profound influence in the life of Essayist 32, and she correctly devotes her theme to the healing power of music and her study of musical therapy. Essays 10, 11, and 18 do not make music the theme of their essays, but they do each mention their talents, making them seem more diverse, with a variety of interests.

Essayist 10 draws a compelling portrait of an avid skier and swimmer and effectively ties her interest in sports to medicine through her experience as a lifeguard and a member of the emergency medical ski team. Essayist 18 mentions learning tennis as a new sport as part of her "participation in activities which have helped me mature as a person."

Students of Diversity

If you are diverse in any sense of the word—an older applicant, a minority, a foreign applicant, or disabled—use it to your advantage by showing what your unique background will bring to the school and to the practice of medicine. Some admissions officers, however, warn against using minority status as a qualification instead of a quality. If you fall into this trap, your diversity will work against you.

If you are a "student of diversity," feel free to discuss it. But don't harp on it for it's own sake or think that being diverse by itself is enough to get you in; that will only make us feel manipulated and it will show that you didn't know how to take advantage of a good opportunity.

So just be sure you tie it in with either your motivation or your argument for why your diversity makes you an interesting candidate.

Latecomers and Career Switchers

You need not be a minority, a foreign applicant, disabled, or an athlete or musician to be considered diverse. There are, for example, those who have had experience in or prepared themselves for totally different fields. Essay 30 was written by a management consultant who was looking to switch careers. Essayist 3 begins by discussing how miserable he was as branch manager for a marketing corporation. Essay 19 was written by a woman who had always planned to go into Public Health, and Essayist 35 originally wanted to be a veterinarian. All of them give succinct reasons for wanting to go into medicine and show evidence of sincere and intensive preparation for their new chosen field.

English Majors and Theater People

Not everyone who is accepted to medical school has a hard-core science background. Essayist 1 originally wanted to be a writer and writes persuasively on the similarities between analyzing literature and analyzing medical research. He takes this one step further when discussing the creative versus the analytical approach to medicine and his lofty ambition of building a bridge between the two. Essay 7 opens with the author's involvement in a play, and she openly admits that she was initially turned off by science and math. Essayist 13 also discusses the writer's late interest in medicine and early preference for the arts. Essayist 22 was a Classics major; Essayist 28 was an Art History major. Essayist 35 admits that she "turned away from science during my undergraduate years" and Essayist 14 mentions that he has been a grammar tutor, editor, and script writer.

The secret of all these essayists is that they know how to turn what may be perceived as weaknesses into strengths. They point out that communication is an integral part of being a doctor, and discuss the advantages of their well-rounded backgrounds. They are also very careful to demonstrate their motivation and qualifications in detail and with solid evidence to offset worries that their liberal arts backgrounds may have given them an unrealistic view of a doctor's life or that they might be unable to cope with the science courses in medical school.

Can I Be Too Well Rounded?

Some people have talents, abilities, or experience in so many different areas that they risk coming across as unfocused or undedicated. When handled deftly, though, your many sides can be brought together, and what could have hurt you becomes instead your greatest vehicle for setting you apart from the crowd. One essayist who does a terrific job of this is the writer of Essay 28. She was an art history major, active in varsity sports, health education, and traveling. After college, she was an au pair in Iceland and an exchange student and intern in France. She manages to present all of this in a short, pointed essay by using the concept of connections as her theme. She relates systems of connections both to the human body as well as to her own diverse activities, emphasizing how they all come together to form a coherent and unique whole. Other essayists who had to deal with their wide range of interests include 12, 13, and 18.

Taking Advantage of International Experience

Many applicants have international experience. So, while it may not set you apart in a completely unique way, it is always worthwhile to demonstrate your cross-cultural experience and sensitivity. Some of the essayists in this book describe fascinating international experience ranging from volunteering in Africa (11), Brazil (21), and Honduras (33), to being an au pair in Iceland (28), to opera singing in Paris (32). Essay 31 is especially strong in the area of international experience. This exceptional man worked as a farmhand in Hungary and an orderly in the former Soviet Union, financed the first hospital in Estonia, and organized a mission to deliver medical supplies to refugees in Bosnia.

Notice again, though, that all these essayists went beyond simply writing about their experiences to relating them either to their motivation or qualifications. Do not expect the committee to make these leaps for you; you need to put it in your own words and make the connections clear.

Religion

Some admissions counselors advise against the mention of religion altogether. Others say that it can be used to applicants' advantage by setting them apart and by stressing values and commitment. This is a sensitive subject area and is best left to individual choice. Essays 13, 18, and 34 all mention religion to varying degrees. The writer of Essay 13 was a missionary for the Church of Jesus Christ of Latter-Day Saints for two years; Essayist 34 is an elder of the same. Essayist 18 mentions Bible study briefly, but it still sheds light on what is probably an important part of her life.

Theme 3: What Your Qualifications and Experiences Are

The last major theme deals with your experience and qualifications both for attending medical school and for becoming a good doctor. Having direct hospital patient care or research experience is always the best evidence you can give. If you have none, then consider what other experience you have that is related. Have you been a volunteer? Have you tutored English as a Second Language? Were you a teaching assistant? The rule to follow here is: If you have done it, use it.

Hospital/Clinical Experience

Direct experience with patients is probably the best kind to have in your essay. But the important thing to remember here is that any type or amount of experience you have had should be mentioned, no matter how insignificant you feel it is. Many of the essayists in this book cited experiences they had in high school. Many were volunteers, some as HIV counselors (16), some in emergency rooms (20, 35), some as lab assistants (29), some as observers (34), and some simply escorted patients to their rooms (5).

Research Experience

A word of caution: Do not focus solely on your research topic; your essay will become impersonal at best and positively dull at worst. Watch out for overuse of what nonscience types refer to as "medical garble." If it is necessary for the description of your project, then, of course, you have no choice. But including medical terms in your essay just because you are able to will not impress anyone. Essayists 14 and 20, for example, delve into the use of scientific and medical terms, but they also spend enough time away from them to reveal their own personal, nontechnical voice.

Unusual Medical Experience

Even if you have not volunteered X number of hours a week at a clinic or spent a term on a research project, you might still have medical experience that counts: the time you cared for your sick grandmother (Essays 2 and 18) or the day you saved the man at the next table from choking in a restaurant. It does not even matter if you were unsuccessful (maybe, despite all your valiant efforts, the man at the next table did not survive); if it was meaningful to you then it is relevant. In fact, these failed efforts might be even more compelling. Essayists 10, 23, and 34 all relay tales of failing to save a life. Essay 33, on the other hand, deals with a fascinating success story: The writer was forced to become a doctor by default in a village in Honduras for a summer, even though she had no formal training, no experience, and her only supply was "a $15 Johnson & Johnson kit."

Nonmedical Experience

Your experience does not even have to be medically related to be relevant. Many successful applicants cite nonmedical volunteer experience as evidence of their willingness to help and heal the human race. In fact, almost every one of our essayists cited having been either a volunteer or a tutor at some point in their lives.

Pitfall Number 2: Making Lists

There is an inherent danger in wanting to cram as much of your experience as possible into 500 words. The danger is in ending up with what amounts to little more than a listing of your accomplishments.

I've found that medical school applicants can have a tendency to make laundry lists. They need to take extra care to tie their interests, motivation, and preparation together and turn it into a readable and credible argument that fits them.

It is not a bad idea to include all the experience you have had somewhere in your essay, but do it in the context of a story or a personal account.

The essay should never be merely a prose form of a C.V. It's dry to read, and again, doesn't offer any additional information about the candidate.

Strategic Tips

Once you have decided which themes to incorporate into your essay, the last step is to develop a strategy; in other words, determine how you will weave your themes together. Here is some advice you do not get often: Don't think about this one too much. The nice thing about strategy is that it tends to fall into place by itself once you develop an outline and start writing, which is what a later chapter is all about. So what we offer here is no more than a couple of tips for you to consider—but not to worry too much about. In the end there really is no more we can tell you about strategy without knowing more about you personally.

Strategy Tip 1: Keep the School in Mind

Most students write generic personal statements that are then sent to every school. That is fine, and to a degree it is expected. But it always impresses a committee when you do your research and show in your essay why you are a good fit for that particular school.

Know the schools to which you are applying and know what they look for in an applicant. Some schools are heavily research-based, some only want in-state residents, some want the heaviest science preparation possible. Do your homework!

Don't be lazy about this! You can, at the very least, find out about the school's general reputation by scanning the guidebook and catalog. However, it is better to research the faculty and familiarize yourself with a school's specific strengths. All of this becomes fodder for the statement and will be crucial later when you are invited to interview.

Essays 25 and 26 are examples of how the same applicant tweaked her essay to work for two different programs. In the first of the two (25), she was applying to (and accepted to) the Harvard MIT Division of Health Sciences and Technology Program and she stresses her analytical skills and computer experience. The second was sent to (and accepted by) Yale, University of Pennsylvania, Johns Hopkins University, and New York University medical schools, and she stresses a more socially minded and humanistic side by describing her volunteer and tutoring work at an after-school literacy program.

Strategy Tip 2: Keep the Rest of Your Application in Mind

Step back and take an objective look at your entire application package. Imagine that you are the admissions officer looking at it for the first time. What do the test scores, the science and nonscience GPA, the kinds of courses you took, the recommendations, the extracurriculars, and the supplementary materials say about you? Do you feel the package presents a complete picture of you? If it doesn't, what can you include in your essay to round it out? Also note if there are any obvious red flags:

> *If there is a hole or gap that appears in another part of the application, we will look to the statement to provide an explanation. If one is not provided, we start guessing. Anything the candidate provides is bound to be better than what we hypothesize in its absence.*

Also note redundancies. Do not recapitulate in your essay those items that can be found elsewhere in the application. Do not repeat your GPA or your MCAT score, no matter how impressive. And, as noted previously, do not try to cram in a prose listing of your activities and accomplishments when space is provided for you to do that elsewhere. Not only is it dull, but it shows that you do not know how to take advantage of a good opportunity to showcase your personal qualities.

Pitfall Number 3: Excuses, Excuses

Because GPAs and MCATs are so important to the application process, applicants who have fallen short in either area are often tempted to use the essay to provide excuses for their poor performances. As previously noted, if there is a true anomaly in your record, the committee will look to your essay for an explanation. Applicants who do this well provide a brief and mature explanation of the lapse, and they spend the rest of the essay focusing on their strengths in other areas.

Explaining a bad grade or even a bad semester can be done with finesse. But, please, just don't whine while you're doing it.

The problems come when an applicant attempts to excuse a problem instead of explaining it. Some applicants, for example, try to excuse a low MCAT score by claiming that they are not good test takers. Well, we hate to break it to them, but medical school involves taking tests. They are a large part of the curriculum and are proven predictors of academic success. So, admitting to being a bad tester would not be a good thing, even if you are being honest. Other students try to push the blame for a bad grade onto someone else.

Using the essay to make excuses for your overall poor record isn't a good way to get ahead. We don't need to hear about the professor who "had a problem with you," or how your organic chemistry professor "wasn't from America." These types of statements speak volumes about a person's character.

The only way to know for sure that you are not falling into this trap is to ask someone objective to proof your essay for you. Even better, find someone who does not even know you and ask that person to describe back to you the impression he or she received of the writer.

Strategy Tip 3: Avoid Discussing Medical Issues

Though known to come up during interviews, a discussion of medical issues is not often attempted in the essay and not generally advised. There are many reasons for this:

1. The essay is supposed to be about you, not about issues.
2. Your audience likely knows more about the issues than you do.
3. With only two pages to do the issue justice, you will probably end up attempting to cover more than you can accomplish.
4. You risk offending someone on the committee. The natural exception to this rule is if a medical issue featured prominently in your decision to become a doctor. Essayist 12, for example, cites the public health care debate as one of her primary draws to the field.

Discussing your negative views of the medical field in your personal statement is an especially risky way to address medical issues. As in anything, there are those who do it well. Essayist 1, for example, discusses what he perceives as a conflict in the medical world and demonstrates how he will contribute to the resolution of the conflict. Though he deals with what he sees as a negative conflict in the medical arena, he discusses it objectively and with tact. The writer of Essay 10 does not give her opinion on medical issues, but she does cite the unpleasant experience she had with her pediatrician as the chief motivation to do a better job as a doctor herself. The writers in both of these examples discuss their potential roles in the resolution of the conflict. Even when you keep these tactics in mind, the best advice here is definitely: When in doubt, leave it out.

An Alternative Approach

No matter how stringent these rules regarding theme and strategy may seem, there will always be applicants who decide to toss it all to the wind and take a completely different approach. The writer of Essay 38, for example, incorporates none of the mentioned themes into his personal statement. He does not talk about his motivation or qualifications for attending medical school. In fact, he only mentions medical school once, and even then it is a single reference made only in passing. He chose, instead, to focus his entire essay on his experience as a rower at Cambridge University in England.

This is a risky approach, and one that is best taken by students with very strong applications. This applicant obviously felt confident that the rest of his application spoke well enough of his qualifications that he could focus entirely on another aspect of his life. And this approach does have the merit of painting a vivid picture of the applicant in his natural surroundings and of giving the reader a strong sense of his character and drive. Ultimately it is a personal decision. Again, the best way to gauge whether or not the risk is one worth taking is by finding a reader capable of giving you objective and informed feedback.

PART THREE

Writing the Essay

Congratulations! You have made it through all the preparatory steps needed to write the best essay possible. Give yourself a pat on the back; you are almost done. "But how can that be possible," you may ask, "when I have not even started writing?"

If you followed all the steps prior to this one, then you should have a clear picture in your mind of what you plan to say and how you plan to say it. All you have to do now is transfer the essay from your mind to the paper. Believe it or not, this step is easier than you think.

Writing is difficult only when you do not know what points you want to make, have not decided which material to use to make your points, or are insecure about your writing skills. If you have been following the tips and exercises in previous parts of this book, then you have addressed the first two potential problems already. The next chapter is designed to help you get past the third. It takes you step by step through the process of actually writing an essay, using plenty of examples along the way. So put your anxieties aside and get ready to write.

At Last, Write!

Highlights
- Creating an outline will help you write a well-structured essay.
- Properly constructed paragraphs are the pillars of the essay.
- Effective transitions between paragraphs are essential to a cohesive essay.
- The lead should grab your reader's attention from the beginning.
- The final sentence should tie together loose ends, summarize, or emphasize your main points.

Do's
- Do use a thesaurus if you are having trouble finding the right word.
- Do choose verbs over adverbs and adjectives as much as possible.

Don'ts
- Don't overuse transitional words (however, nevertheless, furthermore).
- Don't overuse the thesaurus—it will show.
- Don't use sentences that are excessively long or short.

Now that you know what you want your personal statement to say, it's time to start writing. First, set a time limit of no more than a couple of days. The longer your time frame, the more difficult it may be to pull your themes together and to write a truly cohesive essay.

The point is not to allow yourself to sit around waiting for inspiration to strike. As one admissions officer put it, "Some of the worst writing ever crafted has been done under the guise of inspiration."

Relieve some of the pressure of writing by reminding yourself that this is just a draft and rid yourself of the notion that your essay can be perfect on the first try. Don't agonize over a particular word choice, or the phrasing of an idea—you will have plenty of time to perfect the essay later. For now, you just need to start. The most important thing is to *get the words on paper.*

Creating an Outline

You are probably familiar by now with the structure of the traditional outline that you have been using since high school:

Paragraph 1
Introduction that contains the central idea

Paragraph 2
Topic sentence that ties into the central idea
First supporting point
Evidence for point

Paragraph 3
Topic sentence that links the above paragraph to the next
Second supporting point
Evidence for point

Paragraph 4
Topic sentence that links the above paragraph to the next
Third supporting point
Evidence for point

Paragraph 5
Conclusion that reiterates the central idea and takes it one step further

The problem with this simple structure is that it does not allow for the complexities created by the multiple themes that need to be incorporated into a personal statement. Your outline is going to end up looking more complicated than this one, but that is no excuse for not having one. In fact, the more complex the essay, the more critical the outline will be. Without it, your essay will lack structure; without structure, your essay will be rambling, ineffective, and difficult to follow.

To get ideas for some different outlines that could be applied to your statement, look at some of the examples below.

Standard Structure

The standard structure is the most common and is recommended for use in almost any circumstance. Applying it is as close as you can get at this level to the simple structure outlined above. The general application of the standard structure is to introduce the themes and main points in the introduction, use the body of the text to supply one supporting point in each paragraph, and then reiterate your main points in the conclusion in light of the evidence that was presented. The following is an example of a pure standard structure used by an applicant who wanted to make the points that she was both interested in and qualified for the medical field on two levels: intellectually, and from a standpoint of wanting to help people:

Paragraph 1 (Introduction)

Leading sentence: "Since my childhood, my father's inspirational accounts as a cardiologist have captured my heart and my interest."

Summary of main points: Introduces "two fundamental tenets" of "working to care and working to cure," noting her interest in both the academic and the caring sides of medicine.

Paragraph 2

Transition sentence: "During my high school and college years, I have explored different areas of community service."

First supporting point: Interest in caring is shown through her community involvement.

Evidence: Tutoring geometry to high school students and English to recent immigrants.

Paragraph 3

Transition sentence: "I have also participated in the caring element of the medical profession, providing companionship to patients in the hospital setting."

Second supporting point: Interest in caring demonstrated by her hospital experience.

Evidence: Volunteer at several hospitals including the Coronary Care Unit and the Cardiac Rehabilitation Center.

Paragraph 4

Transition sentence: "It would be simplistic for me to say that I have chosen to devote my life to the medical profession only because I have a strong desire to help people."

Second supporting point: Also motivated by intellectual exploration.

Evidence: She details her passion for "[making] an intellectual leap and [managing] to land feet first upon a convincing conclusion" and describes the thrill that leaves her "thirsting for the next challenge."

Paragraph 5

Transition sentence: "The excitement of intellectual discovery has encouraged me to explore a number of fields."

Second supporting point: Has a well-rounded academic background.

Evidence: "While my major is biochemistry, my academic interests also encompass Asian studies, languages, music, computer science, health care, and environmental policy. . ."

Paragraph 6

Transition sentence: "My rewarding experiences in growing intellectually have not only fueled my own passion for exploration and discovery, but have inspired me to share my enthusiasm for learning with others, particularly in the field of science."

Second supporting point: Ties academic interests back into the original theme of caring for people.

Evidence: "To help high school students embark on their own exciting voyages to understand the world around us, I wrote a study guide describing how to approach scientific research and titled it *Frontier* to emphasize exploration and intellectual discovery."

Paragraph 7 (Conclusion)

Transition sentence: "To me, there is only one profession which satisfies both my curiosity and my desire to help those in need."

Reiteration of main points and closing sentence: "Incorporating both the caring, personal, physician-patient relationship and the dynamism of continuous learning, the medical profession is the profession I eagerly embrace, and I believe it is also the best way I can harness my own talents and abilities for the benefit of others."

Compare/Contrast

Not all applicants choose the traditional standard structure for their personal statement. The writer of Essay 6 chose to structure his essay, for example, around a comparison between music and medicine:

Paragraph 1 (Introduction)

Leading sentence: "The beating of an African healing drum resonates throughout all corners of the Catholic church during the weekly five o'clock student mass."

The sentence gives a description of the congregation responding to the music he provides at Mass.

Paragraph 2

Transition sentence: "While a drumming performance in church may appear a little unorthodox, the concept of rhythm has never seemed very offbeat to me."

In this sentence he introduces himself and his love of music.

Evidence: Many years of drum lessons, the development of his personal style, the success of his rock band, and the production of a CD.

Paragraph 3

Transition sentence: "Concurrently, my passion for science began to crystallize."

Here he introduces his love for science and medicine.

Evidence: He won a science fair award, volunteered in an emergency room, tutored science and math, and worked in a cancer research laboratory.

Paragraph 4 (Conclusion)

Transition sentence: "It has become clear that the most attractive features to me in the diverse fields of science and music are one and the same."

He concludes with a comparison between his two themes.

Evidence: Both are an exercise in expression and communication . . .

Closing sentence: "I know that my concept of the rhythm of life will help keep me grounded in the fundamentals as I strive to convey and apply my knowledge and gifts to others."

Chronology

Another way to create an outline of your essay is by retelling the events of your life chronologically. The advantage of this approach is that its allows for a more personal approach and helps the committee to know you by turning the focus to you throughout various stages of your life. The drawback is that the points you are trying to make can get lost in the narration of your life.

The writer of Essay 13 uses a chronological structure beginning with the clip of an article describing him as a young boy:

Paragraph 1 (Leading quote)
> *Leading sentence:* "One time, a family cat captured . . . a moth."
> This sentence provides a quote from an article describing him as a boy in 1978.

Paragraph 2 (Introduction)
> *Transition sentence:* "This article, about me as a ten-year-old boy trying to turn a nearby drainage pond into a park, had a misprint—it was a mouse, not a moth."
> This explains the quote and makes the main point that he was cut out to be a doctor from a young age.

Paragraph 3
> *Transition sentence:* "We didn't exactly live on a farm, but were in farming country."
> Here he describes himself and his life as a boy.

Paragraph 4
> *Transition sentence:* "During this period, we did manage to find time for other things."
> Here the writer focuses on his multiple activities throughout his high school years.

Paragraph 5
> *Transition sentence:* "After two semesters at Boise State, I volunteered to serve for two years as a missionary with the Church of Jesus Christ of Latter-Day Saints, going to the California, Ventura Mission."
> The writer continues on to his college years spent as a missionary.

Paragraph 6
> *Transition sentence:* "Returning to school, my classes included math and sciences (subjects I had shied away from before)—out of curiosity, at first; then, to keep my options open."
> He progresses to his return to college and his activities and accomplishments from that period.

Paragraph 7
> *Transition sentence:* "In high school, I had had some health problems and had seen a number of doctors."
> The writer goes back to his high school experiences to introduce the theme of medicine.

Paragraph 8
> *Transition sentence:* "This experience soured me on the medical profession."
> Here he interprets experiences described in the last paragraph to explain his late interest in medicine.

Paragraph 9

Transition sentence: "I pursued psychology and the humanities, while growing more fascinated by health, nutrition, and what people I knew had found in 'alternative' approaches to health, including preventive and Eastern medicine."

The writer talks about his subsequent interest in fields peripheral to medicine.

Paragraph 10

Transition sentence: "Upon transferring to USC, I found that my view of the medical establishment wasn't really accurate—there ARE those who care more about helping people than about the money or their intellectual pride."

He describes how his interest in medicine solidified while at USC.

Paragraph 11 (Conclusion)

Transition sentence: "Throughout my college career, I have had to support myself financially."

The writer uses the transition to discuss the many jobs he has held throughout the various stages in his life.

Incorporating the Narrative

Beginning your essay with a story is a common and effective method for catching and keeping the reader's interest. This is also a good way to structure your essay if you want to focus on a single event in your life. In its purest form, a narrative essay does nothing but tell the story. It begins and ends with the action. This is not recommended for a personal statement, simply because at some point the connection needs to be drawn from the story to your motivation and qualifications for attending medical school.

The following are some examples of excerpts where writers have incorporated narrative into their essays. Notice how each writer provides a clear transition to the rest of the essay:

Essay 17: The writer begins with a story of working as a deckhand for the Sea Education Association (SEA). He uses the story to demonstrate teamwork skills and the importance of community. He transitions from the story with: "Both at sea and on land, I have found great pleasure in the rewards of upholding and enriching the worlds of which I am a part."

Essay 16: This writer tells the story of her high school teacher's battle with AIDS. Transitions with: "I entered college, believing that biology could explain to me why life's processes went awry."

Essay 30: This writer tells the story of unraveling the past of a prehistoric woman by analyzing her bones and transitions in the last paragraph with: "To a large extent, my choice to become a physician is rooted in my desire to continue to work with the human body. But I want to work with the living."

Essay 34: He incorporates the story of his attempt to save a life aboard a train in Italy into the middle of his essay rather than at the beginning. He uses it to illustrate the lessons he learned of self-forgetful devotion and the importance of attention to detail.

Notice the variety of circumstances to which this type of essay can be applied when comparing these essays. A narrative can span a lifetime or a moment. It does not have to be filled with Hollywood-style action to hold interest. The briefest and simplest of events can take on meaning when told effectively. What makes all of these essays effective is their use of detail, description, and direction.

Structuring the Paragraphs

Paragraphs are the pillars of the essay; they uphold and support the structure. Each one that you write should ideally express a single theme and should have a clear beginning, middle, and end. The beginning should be the sentence that introduces the theme and unless it is the first sentence of the essay, it should also create a smooth transition from the paragraph that preceded it and effectively introduce the new topic. The middle should be composed of supporting sentences central to the main theme of the paragraph. The end, or the final sentence, should be a strong conclusion that ties the preceding thoughts together. You should attempt to compose each paragraph of no less than three sentences.

Look at Essay 36 for an example of what is meant by writing solid paragraphs. The essay is made up of six paragraphs. Notice that each one contains a single theme introduced by a topic sentence and supported by concrete evidence or imagery.

Paragraph 1

Introduction. Begins: "Why on Earth do you want to study in Africa?" This writer introduces the essay by describing her experience studying for three months in Kenya.

Paragraph 2

First point. Begins: "A career in medicine appears to be a lot like studying in Kenya." The writer supports the point by comparing a description of her work in Kenya with a medicine career.

Paragraph 3

Second point. Begins: "My first encounter with medical science was as a Women in Science Project Intern in the Norris Cotton Cancer Center of the Dartmouth-Hitchcock Medical Center." She describes her experience there, what she learned, and why it motivated her.

Paragraph 4

Third point. Begins: "In addition to my enthusiasm for science, I have a deep-rooted interest in art history." Briefly discusses her art hobby and why it will provide balance to her primary interest of medicine.

Paragraph 5

Fourth point. Begins: "However, both my research experiences and my study of art have left me devoid of the satisfaction of helping people that I felt throughout high school and college, working directly with several community service organizations." The essayist provides backup and evidence by describing numerous volunteer and tutoring experiences. She ties this experience back to her motivation to be a doctor.

Paragraph 6

Conclusion. Transitions with: "A career as a physician would unite my excitement for learning and my desire for helping others into a distinct whole." The writer closes with a reiteration of her desire to attend and her qualifications for medical school.

Creating Effective Transitions

As you can see from all the examples used so far in this chapter, the first sentences of every paragraph are extremely important. They uphold the structure of your essay and help create strong, targeted paragraphs. They also serve as transitions linking your points together. An essay without good transitions is just a group of unrelated thoughts. The reader will struggle to get from one point to the next. Use transitions as bridges between your ideas.

The transition into the final paragraph is especially critical. If it is not clear how you arrived at this final idea, you have either shoehorned a conclusion into the outline, or your outline lacks focus. You should not have to think too much about consciously constructing transitional sentences. If the concepts in your outline follow and build on one another naturally, transitions will practically write themselves. To make sure that you are not forcing them, try to refrain from using words such as: *however, nevertheless,* and *furthermore.*

If you are having trouble transitioning between paragraphs, or are trying to force a transition onto a paragraph that has already been written, it may be indicative of a problem with your structure. If you suspect this to be the case, go back to your original outline and make sure that you have assigned only one point to each paragraph, and that each point naturally follows the preceding one and leads to a logical conclusion. This may result in a kind of back-to-the-drawing-board restructuring, but try not to get frustrated. This happens to even the most seasoned writers and is a normal part of the writing process.

Choosing the Right Words

Well-structured outlines, paragraphs, and transitions are all an important part of creating a solid essay. But structure isn't everything. An essay can be very well organized with balanced paragraphs and smooth transitions and still come across as dull and uninspired. You know from a previous chapter that details are integral to interesting essays. While adding detail is certainly a good start, there is more to know about the kind of writing that holds a reader's attention. First, there is word choice.

Rule 1: Use your thesaurus sparingly

It won't necessarily make you appear smarter; instead, it could make you look as though you are *trying* to *appear* smarter. The overuse of a thesaurus can be dangerous because it is often spotted easily. The last thing you want is for the admissions committee to envision you with a dictionary in one hand and a thesaurus in the other as you craft your personal statement. This will only serve to undermine your writing skills.

However, if it is a simple word choice that you are struggling with or if you find yourself repeating the same word in one sentence or in consecutive sentences, then a thesaurus can actually serve as a useful tool. Similarly, if you aren't sure if a particular word is exactly right in conveying your thoughts, first look it up. If it is not spot on, then a thesaurus may be helpful in finding the perfect word.

Rule 2: Focus on verbs

Try to focus on verb usage instead of relying too heavily on adjectives and adverbs. Pumping your sentences full of adjectives and adverbs is not the same as adding detail or color. They certainly add description, but verbs add action, and action is often more interesting than description.

Composing Proper Sentences

If you are unsure if your sentences are too short or too long, try reading your essay aloud either to yourself, or if possible, to someone else. If you find that you have to pause and take a breath between one period and the next, or if your reader lets out a "Whoa, slow down. . .what was that again?" your sentences may be too long. On the other hand, if you feel that you are taking too many pauses and that the essay sounds a bit choppy, your sentences may be too short.

The risk of having sentences that are too long is that you overwhelm your reader or that you lose them all together. If the reader has to stop reading and start again because your sentences are too wordy, you have either not provided adequate punctuation, or more likely, you have rambled on too long. There are a few ways to go back and correct this. First, make sure you've used sufficient (and correct) punctuation. Commas and semicolons can be an absolute necessity in long sentences. If punctuation alone doesn't do the trick, look for an overuse of adjectives and adverbs. While descriptive words can be fantastic in creating imagery for your reader, if used too often or if too many are crammed together in succession, they can just create a jumbled mess. If you've inserted a lot of commas just to correctly punctuate your descriptions, you've probably used too many adjectives and/or adverbs. Try to simplify your descriptions using fewer but more effective words. Finally, if you haven't already done so, break the longer sentences up into shorter sentences that flow after one another smoothly and logically.

A bit less risky but still worth noting are short, choppy sentences. If you find that most of your sentences are no more than a few words, you may have written an essay that is not descriptive enough and that lacks fluidity. Remember that your sentences, not just your paragraphs, need to transition smoothly from one to the next and many of them need to support those that preceded them.

Writing Introductions and Conclusions

Beginnings and endings can be the most challenging part of crafting any piece of writing—and also, in many ways, the most important. Part of the reason they are so difficult is that writers tend to worry about them so much. There is so much hype about the necessity of thoroughly introducing the subject and ending with sharply drawn conclusions that anxious essayists compensate by going overboard. They feel that in order to appear mature and worldly their essays must contain profound insights and sweeping observations.

Do not fall into this trap! One of the biggest complaints that our admissions officers had was that essayists tried to say and do too much in their introductions. "Just tell the story!" wrote one officer repeatedly in response to numerous essays.

Formal Introductions

If you are able to construct seamless introductions and conclusions as soon as your pen hits the paper, you are way ahead of the game. However, if you are having trouble, do not let it impede the writing process. You still need to get your thoughts on paper so don't worry about crafting effective beginnings and endings at this point. Just dive in and see where your pen leads you. You may find that compelling beginnings and endings write themselves. Especially if your essay begins with a story or a quote, you may find that a formal introduction isn't required. If your style is on the creative side, not having a traditional introduction may actually work just fine. However, if your essay follows the standard format, you can always go back and work on the introductions and conclusions, or the beginnings and endings, when you've gotten the bulk of your thoughts on paper. You may even find that it is easier this way.

Leading the Way

The most important part of any beginning is, of course, the lead. Leads play the dual role of setting the theme of your essay and engaging the reader. The introduction should not be overly formal. You do not want an admissions officer to start reading your essay and think, "Here we go again." Although admissions officers will try to give the entire essay a fair reading, they are only human; if you lose them after the first sentence, the rest of your essay will not get the attention it deserves.

Just as you should not worry about your introduction until you have gotten an initial draft on paper, you should not begin by writing your lead. Often, you will spot a good one floating around in the middle of your first draft of the essay, so don't worry about it until you have the bulk of your essay on paper.

There are many different kinds of effective leads. You will find examples of some of them listed below.

Standard Lead

Standard leads are the most common leads used. A typical standard lead answers one or more of the six basic questions: *who, what, when, where, why*, and *how*. They give the reader an idea of what to expect. A summary lead is a kind of standard lead that answers most of these questions in one sentence. The problem with this kind of lead is that, although it is a logical beginning, it can be dull. The advantage is that it sets your reader up for a focused and well-structured essay. If you live up to that expectation, the impact of your points is heightened. They are also useful for shorter essays when you need to get to the point quickly.

> *Initially, my interest in medicine was due to my family.* (Essay 24)

> *I am interested in participating in the Harvard MIT Division of Health Sciences and Technology Program (HST) in the context of an M.D./Ph.D. to prepare for a career in medical research.* (Essay 25)

> *My work experiences—ranging from public health projects in rural Latin America to work at urban battered women's shelters to peer counseling on a college campus—reflect my concern for people's "health" in a broad sense of the word.* (Essay 18)

Creative Lead

This lead attempts to add interest by being obtuse or funny. It may leave the reader wondering what the rest of the essay will be about, but it often serves to spark the interest of the reader right from the beginning—which is always a good thing. If your essay is toward the bottom of a stack of 40 to be read by one person in one day, we think the creative lead may help break the monotony for the reader. You must make it relevant to the text that follows, but when done well, it can lead to a more interesting and, for lack of a better word, *creative* essay.

> *The melody starts low, a quiet whirring sound of violins slowly envelops the hall.* (Essay 32)

> *The beating of an African healing drum resonates throughout all corners of the Catholic church during the weekly five o'clock student mass.* (Essay 6)

> *When I consider my life experiences, I imagine them as a system of bones and joints, interconnected, cooperative, and form-giving.* (Essay 28)

Action Lead

This lead takes the reader into the middle of a piece of action. It is perfect for short essays where space needs to be conserved or for narrative essays that begin with a story.

The car swerved to the left. (Essay 27)

She dropped the box on the table and left the room because she didn't want to watch. (Essay 35)

It was opening night. I was about to walk on stage as Ruth in "The Pirates of Penzance." (Essay 7)

As the rusted-out Land Rover made its way cautiously through dense thicket and crevices in the rocky dirt road, those of us sitting on top were able to peer through the trees at a sublime West African landscape. (Essay 11)

One day in the summer after my graduation from high school, my grandfather took me up to the attic of his house to show me something he thought would be significant for me. (Essay 22)

Personal or Revealing Lead

This lead reveals something about the writer. It is always in the first person and usually takes an informal, conversational tone.

I was not in control of my life and I was miserable. (Essay 3)

Since my childhood, my father's inspirational accounts as a cardiologist have captured my heart and my interest. (Essay 21)

I decided that I wanted to be a doctor some time after my four month incarceration in Columbia Presbyterian Children's Hospital in the winter of 1986-87, as I struggled with anorexia nervosa. (Essay 33)

Quotation Lead

This type of lead can be a direct quotation or a paraphrase. It is most effective when the quote you choose is unusual, funny, or obscure, and not too long. Choose a quote with a meaning you plan to reveal to the reader as the essay progresses. Some admissions officers caution against using this kind of lead because it can seem like you are trying to impress them or sound smart. Do not use a proverb or cliché, and do not interpret the quote in your essay. The admissions committee is more interested in how you respond to it and what that response says about you.

Dr. Lewis Thomas described medicine as "The Youngest Science" because insightful discoveries in basic research have led to revolutionary innovations in clinical therapy that have improved the quality of life. (Essay 5)

"One day you will read in the National Geographic of a faraway land with no smelly bad traffic. In those green-pastured mountains of Fotta-fa-Zee everybody feels fine at a hundred and three 'cause the air that they breathe is potassium-free and because they chew nuts from the Tutt-a-Tutt Tree. This gives strength to their teeth, it gives length to their hair, and they live without doctors, with nary a care."
—*Dr. Seuss, You're Only Old Once* (Essay 10)

I love the way he makes me laugh. (Essay 4)

As a quote is often less naturally applicable to the text that follows than other types of leads, you must be even more conscious of its relevance and your ability to make it work for the essay. If you are at all uncertain with your ability to pull it off, we do not advise using this method because if not done well, it will seem like a gimmick.

Dialogue Lead

This lead takes the reader into a conversation. It can take the form of an actual dialogue between two people or can simply be a snippet of personal thought. It is similar to creative and action leads in that it often serves as the introduction of a story. Similar rules apply when using this type of lead.

"Power ten, next stroke!" shouts the coxswain over the speaker system. (Essay 38)

"Dawn, do you believe in las brujas?" (Essay 19)

"Carl, the woman we're about to meet will receive her first palliative treatment today." (Essay 20)

"Why on Earth do you want to study in Africa?" (Essay 36)

Informative Lead

This lead gives the reader a fact or a statistic that is connected to the topic of your essay or simply provides a piece of information about yourself or a situation. It can be a compelling way to open your essay.

Every doctor remembers his first patient. (Essay 23)

In communist Hungary in 1986 ownership of property meant certain things. (Essay 31)

On the corner of 168th Street and Broadway in New York City there always seems to be a line of people. (Essay 37)

Closing Your Case

The final sentence or two of your essay is also critical. It must conclude your argument or theme, and it is an important part of creating a positive and memorable image. Endings are the last experience an admissions officer has with your essay, so you need to make those words and thoughts count. A standard close merely summarizes the main points you have made.

Some examples of standard closes include:

As a lifelong commitment to society, the medical profession most completely encompasses my career goals and moral values. (Essay 5)

Reminiscing about how M. pulled the browned marshmallow from his chopstick, I am thankful to my campers and students, their families, and my friends for helping me to affirm that this is the path I wish my life to follow. (Essay 8)

If you have introduced a clever or unusual thought in the first paragraph, try referring back to it in your conclusion. The aim is for the admissions officer to leave your essay thinking, "That was a satisfying read," and "I wish there were more."

Essay 27, for example, closes with:

> *The once bewildered seven-year-old at the scene of an accident now has the skills and maturity to do more than change diapers; she aspires to read the film of the broken humerus or to set the cast some day soon.*

This writer's reference to the bewildered seven-year-old relates back to her opening story about a car accident from her youth. This stylistic touch nicely wraps up the essay and shows that time was spent in planning and structuring.

Taking a Break

You have made it through the first draft, and you deserve a reward for the hard work—take a break. Let it sit for a couple of days. You need to distance yourself from the piece so you can gain objectivity. Writing can be an emotional and exhausting process, particularly when you write about yourself and your experiences. After you finish your first draft, you may think a bit too highly of your efforts, or you may be too harsh. Both extremes are probably inaccurate. Once you have let your work sit for awhile, you will be better able to take the next (and final!) step: Making It Perfect.

Making It Perfect

Highlights

- It is constructive to take a break from your essay before beginning the first revision.
- The first revision should focus on content and structure.
- Reading aloud to detect awkward language or phrasing can be effective.
- Eliminating the use of passive voice can strengthen the quality of your essay.
- Grammatical and spelling errors are unacceptable.
- Get feedback!

Writing is not a one-time act. Writing is a process, and memorable writing may come more from rewriting than it does from the first draft. By rewriting, you will improve your essay—guaranteed. There is no perfect number of drafts that will insure a great essay, but you will eventually reach a point when your confidence in the strength of your writing is reinforced by the thoughts of others. If you skimp on the rewriting process, you significantly reduce the chances that your essay will be as good as it can be. Don't take that chance. The following steps show you how to take your essay from rough to remarkable.

Revise

Once you have spent a little time away from your essay, come back and read it with fresh eyes. Analyze it as objectively as possible based on the following three components: substance, structure, and interest. Do not worry yet about surface errors and spelling mistakes; focus instead on the larger issues. Be prepared to find

57

some significant problems with your essays and be willing to address them even though it might mean significantly more work. Also, if you find yourself unable to smooth out the problems that turn up, you should be willing to start from scratch, potentially with a new topic.

Substance

Substance refers to the content of your essay and the message you are sending out. It can be very hard to gauge in your own writing. One good way to make sure that you are saying what you think you are saying is to write down, briefly and in your own words, the message you are trying to communicate. Then remove the introduction and conclusion from your essay and have an objective reader review what is left. Compare the two statements to see how similar they are. This can be especially helpful if you wrote a narrative, to make sure that your points are being communicated in the story.

Here are some more questions to ask yourself regarding content:

- If a specific question was asked, have you answered it?
- Is each point that you make backed up by an example?
- Are your examples concrete and personal?
- Have you been specific? Go on a generalities hunt. Turn the generalities into specifics.
- Is the essay about you? (The answer should be "Yes!")
- What does it say about you? Try making a list of all the words you have used to describe yourself (directly or indirectly). Does the list accurately represent you?
- Does the writing sound like you? Is it personal and informal rather than uptight or stiff?
- Read your introduction. Is it personal and written in your own voice? If it is general or makes any broad claims, then have someone proofread your essay once without it. Did the reader notice that it was missing? If the essay can stand on its own without it, then consider removing it permanently.

Structure

To check the overall structure of your essay, do a first-sentence check. Write down the first sentence of every paragraph in order. Read through them one after another, and ask yourself the following:

- Would someone who was reading only these sentences still understand exactly what you are trying to say?

- Are all of your main points expressed in the first sentences?

- Do the thoughts flow naturally, or do they seem to skip around or come out of left field?

Now go back to your essay as a whole and ask yourself:

- Does each paragraph stick to the thought that was introduced in the first sentence?

- Is each point supported by a piece of evidence? How well does the evidence support the point?

- Is each paragraph of roughly the same length? When you step back and squint at your essay, do the paragraphs look balanced on the page? If one is significantly longer than the rest, you are probably trying to squeeze more than one thought into it.

- Does your conclusion draw naturally from the previous paragraphs?

Interest

Many people think only of mechanics when they revise and rewrite their compositions. But as we know, making your statement interesting is crucial in keeping the admissions officers reading and in making your essay memorable. Look at your essay with the interest equation in mind: personal + specific = interesting. Answer the following:

- Is the opening paragraph personal? Do you start with action or an image?

- At what point does your essay *really* begin? Try to delete all the sentences before that point.

- Does the essay "show" rather than "tell?" Use details whenever possible to create images.

- Did you use any words that you wouldn't use in a conversation? If so, you might consider different language.

- Have you used an active voice? (See more under "The Hunt for Red Flags," following.)

- Are your verbs active and interesting?

- Have you overused adjectives and adverbs?

- Have you eliminated trite expressions and clichés?

- Does it sound interesting to you? If it bores you, it will bore others.

- Will the ending give the reader a sense of completeness? Does the last sentence sound like the conclusion?

The Hunt for Red Flags

How can you know if you are writing in a passive or active voice? Certain words and phrases are red flags for the passive voice, and relying on them too heavily will considerably weaken an otherwise good essay. To find out if your essay is suffering from passivity, go on a hunt for all of the following, highlighting each one as you find it:

really	rather
there is	it is important to note that
it is essential that	however
nonetheless/nevertheless	in addition
in conclusion	for instance
yet	very
although	in fact
I feel	I believe
I hope	can be
maybe	perhaps
usually	may/may not
have had	somewhat

How much of your essay is highlighted? You do not need to eliminate these phrases completely, but ask yourself if each one is necessary. Try replacing the phrase with a stronger one. At times, particularly when writing about a subjective topic, the passive voice can be appropriate. It can cushion the way you describe a personal belief so as not to seem rigid in your thinking, or brash in your assertions. To help determine "how much is OK," use the Read Out Loud technique described on the next page to guide you. In speech, you will likely hear passive phrasing reduce the impact of your statements, and can turn your assertions into mere suggestions. Used excessively, passive speech can weaken the overall credibility of what you are trying to convey.

Proofread

When you are satisfied with the structure and content of your essay, it is time to check for grammar, spelling, typos, and the like. Take advantage of an easy "spelling and grammar check" on your computer. After correcting everything that your software program brings to your attention, go back in and check for issues that it won't find. Keep rewriting until your words say what you want them to say. Ask yourself these questions:

- Did I punctuate correctly?

- Did I end any sentences with prepositions? (The answer should be "No!")

- Did I use excessively long or short sentences?

- Did I eliminate exclamation points (except in dialogue)?

- Do I use capitalization clearly and consistently?

- Do the subjects agree in number with the verbs?

- Did I place the periods and commas inside the quotation marks?

- Did I keep contractions to a minimum? Are apostrophes in the right places?

- Did I replace the name of the proper school for each new application?

Read Out Loud

To help you polish the essay even further, read it out loud. You will be amazed at the faulty grammar and awkward language that your ears can detect. It will also give you a good sense of the flow of the piece and will alert you to anything that sounds too abrupt or out of place. Good writing, like good music, has a certain rhythm. How does your essay sound: interesting and varied, or drawn out and monotonous? Reading out loud is also a good way to catch errors that your eyes might otherwise skim over while reading silently.

Get Feedback

We've mentioned this point many times throughout this book, but it can never be emphasized enough: Get feedback! Not only will it help you see your essay objectively, as others will see it, but it is also a good way to become reinspired when you feel yourself burning out.

You should have already found someone to proof for general style, structure, and content as was advised previously. If you have to write multiple essays for one school, have the set as a whole evaluated. As a final step before submitting your application, find someone new to proof for the surface errors with fresh eyes.

And, as was said earlier, if you are having trouble finding someone willing (and able) to dedicate the time and thought that needs to be put in to make this step effective, you may want to consider getting a professional evaluation. In addition to our own web site (*www.Ivyessays.com*) a number of these types of services can be found on the Internet.

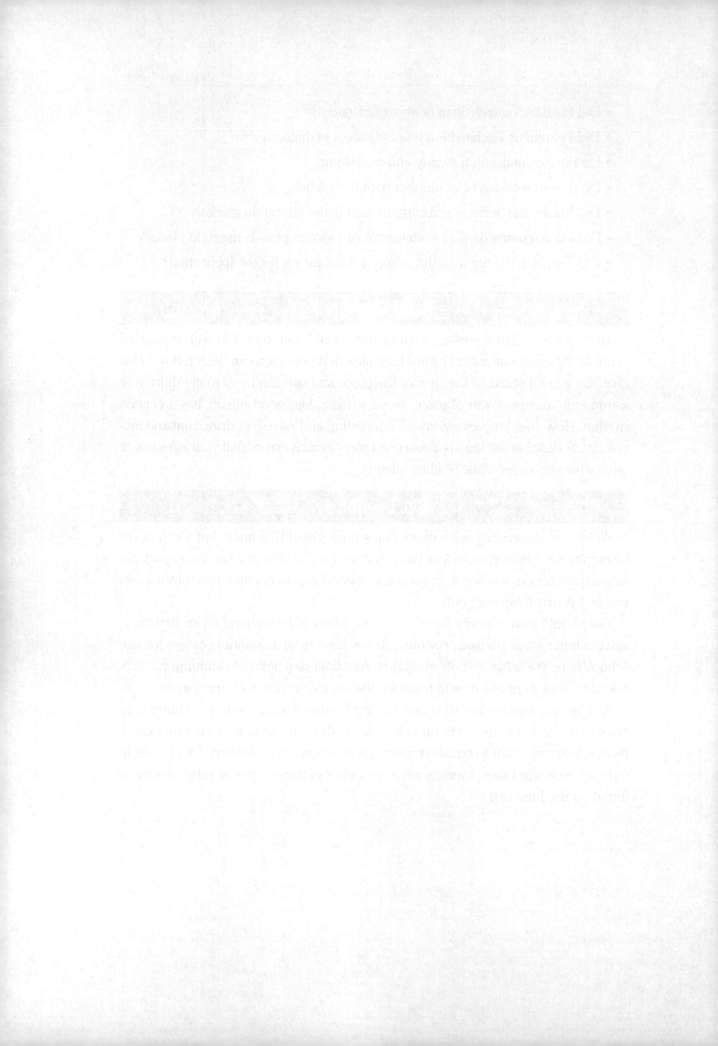

PART FOUR

The Interview

After the first stage of evaluation, once the admissions committee has read the essays and tabulated the numbers, an applicant may be invited to interview. At most schools this is a necessary prerequisite to your acceptance. The percentage of applicants interviewed varies from school to school, and can fall anywhere from 15 percent to 50 percent, based largely on the number of completed applications a given school receives. Perhaps more significant is the percentage of interviewees that are accepted. Again, percentages vary widely by schools but for around 150 spots, many schools estimated interviewing around 1000 applicants. Some were a bit more selective in the number of students invited for interviews, which increased the percentage of interviewees who were admitted. Regardless of how it is broken down, we don't need to convince you at this stage of the game that it is a competitive process.

With this level of competition, the committee has no choice but to look beyond the test scores and other numbers to an applicant's "soft" skills. This is why the interview and the personal statement are both so crucial in the medical admissions process. This chapter will help you prepare for your interview, and answer some key questions about the process: What makes the medical school interview different from a college interview? What are the different kinds of interviews and interview tactics commonly employed by medical admissions teams? What is the best way to prepare?

Preparing for the Interview

Highlights

- Interview formats vary from school to school. To avoid surprise, it may be prudent to research what type of interview you can expect before your scheduled interview.
- Be prepared for your interview: Know everything that is contained in your application and essay, think of how you would answer common interview questions, and have questions prepared to ask the interviewer.
- Try to relax and be yourself.

Do's

- Do research each school that you will visit for an interview.
- Do take it slow and consider your responses.
- Do be completely honest.
- Do research current medical "hot topics" and be ready to discuss them.
- Do know where you stand on ethical medical issues.
- Do dress professionally.
- Do act respectful, interested, focused, and attentive.
- Do write thank-you notes to each interviewer.

Don'ts

- Don't arrive late, tired, or overly anxious.
- Don't say "um" or "like" any more than you can possibly help it.
- Don't repeat or contradict yourself.
- Don't try to be someone you are not.
- Don't fidget, chew gum, or take food or drink into the interview.

The medical school interview is a little different from the college-level interview or a typical job interview. For example, it is more competitive in that acceptance-to-interview ratios are probably lower than other interviews you have had. Also, you could face multiple interviews in one day and possibly multiple interviewers in one session. Finally, the interviewers are M.D.s, Ph.D.s, and medical students. They are experts on medicine, but not always experts at interviewing. The implications of this can be harrowing, but there are strategies you can learn to make it easier. If you prepare yourself well, you can enter the interview process confidently, and that alone is half the battle.

Types of Interviews

The type of interview you will encounter will be different at every medical school. Pick and choose from any of the following variables:

MORE COMMON	LESS COMMON
You are interviewed by one person.	You are interviewed by a committee.
You are interviewed once.	You are interviewed several times.
You are interviewed by a faculty member or student.	You are interviewed by a member of the admissions staff or a community doctor.
You are the only interviewee.	You are interviewed with a group of applicants.
The interviewer is familiar with your file and background and has prepared specific questions for you.	The interviewer comes to the interview completely unfamiliar with your background or qualifications.
The interviewer is relaxed and conversational.	The interviewer is formal and structured and grills you on your knowledge and qualifications.

To eliminate some of the guesswork before you arrive at the interview, some admissions officers say that it is OK to call ahead and ask for the names of your interviewers and whether they are faculty, students, or whatever. You can take this a step further by researching the interviewers personally (for instance, what have they published, what courses they teach, are they M.D.s or Ph.D.s, and so on). Other admissions officers advised against taking this step, and cautioned that schools will often withhold this information to avoid calls to the interviewer and because emergencies can cause the interviewers to change at the last minute.

Tips for Interviewing Successfully

Tip 1: Do Your Homework

There is a commonly held misconception that there is no real way to prepare for an interview. This is absolutely untrue. No matter what type of interview you have, whether it is inquisitive or conversational, being prepared is the secret to success. You must be prepared to talk intelligently about the two most important pieces in the application puzzle—yourself and the school.

1. **Look at your entire application objectively.** What impressions or preconceptions would you have about the person described? Do you see any areas of potential weakness? Are there any red flags that need explaining? Make a list of the kinds of questions that you would ask someone with your background, then practice answering them out loud.

2. **Reread your essay.** A lot of interviewers focus on the essay or use it as the icebreaker. Look at it objectively and try to imagine what more you would want to know about the writer. Be ready to discuss in depth anything you've written about or even mentioned in the personal statement. If your interview and your personal statement don't back each other up, you will come across as insincere, or worse, dishonest.

3. **Think of some key points that you want to communicate to the interviewer.** Practice making these points out loud. Think of ways to incorporate your points into answers to open-ended questions.

4. **Practice answering common interview questions.** You will find a list of these questions in the next chapter. Develop thorough and precise answers for each question type, and think about the different experiences you could talk about to demonstrate each point you would like to make.

5. **Prepare a list of questions you want to ask the interviewers.** Have enough questions that you aren't forced to ask the same questions of different interviewers in case they compare notes. You shouldn't ask questions just because it's expected, and don't go overboard by asking too many. Take the time to think of the questions that shed further light on what is important to you. Pick and choose from the next chapter the questions that are most relevant to you.

6. **Prepare to answer, as well as ask, questions about the school.** Refer back to the research you did earlier for your essay. What were the features that drew you to the school? Select key points and criteria, and then prepare your questions. Demonstrate your knowledge of the school and the level of your commitment to it. Think of questions that address your long-term goals and how the school's program ties into them.

7. **Prepare to talk about current medical issues.** It is very common for an interviewer to touch on at least one hot topic. Many of these types of questions will pose ethical dilemmas. Where you stand on the issue probably won't matter as much as your ability to demonstrate your familiarity with it and your ability to discuss it intelligently. Some current medical issues that would be prudent to brush up on would be stem cell research, cloning, and universal healthcare. Some long-standing ethical dilemmas in the field could lead to questions about your feelings toward abortion, euthanasia, and research on human and animal subjects. If you stay current with at least one popular medical journal, you will probably be able to tackle most questions that could be posed.

Tip 2: Relax

If you've done all the above preparation, than there is only one thing left for you to do to ensure a successful interview: Relax! You should look at it as an opportunity to exchange opinions, information, and views. Interviewers are people. They all endured the same process, and they understand how you feel. Also, don't forget that you are evaluating them too. You are both on the stage together, and some of the control belongs to you.

Still nervous? Review your notes again. Practice some more. Take deep breaths. Take your time before answering each question. Intentionally speak at a slower pace and lower tone than you would ordinarily (we speak faster and our pitch rises when we're nervous). Imagine that you are talking to a friend. In short, do whatever you can do to keep your nerves at a manageable pitch. A little anxiety is fine; it is natural and can help make you seem animated in the interview.

Tip 3: Be Yourself

As with your essay, don't try to be something you are not in the interview—it will show. Be honest, sincere, and truthful. Don't say you've done things you haven't done, read books you haven't read, or are interested in things you are not. And whatever you do, don't lie about your grades or test scores. Show them who you are with specific examples from your life.

Give them your heartfelt opinion, even when they ask you the difficult questions about medical issues or health care reform plans. They're not looking for your opinion so much as how you present it: Have you put some thought into your answer? Are you up on current medical issues? Is your thinking logical and well reasoned? Are you ethically motivated? Admissions officers consider an interview successful when they walk away feeling that they've met the real you; it doesn't matter if the two of you disagree on an issue.

The Failproof Fallback Plan

No matter how thoroughly you've prepared, someone will always find a way to throw you a curveball. At some point you will likely be faced with a question you were not expecting, one that doesn't fit any of your prepared points. What then?

Don't panic. Ironically, not being able to answer a question is often a result of being *over*prepared rather than *un*prepared. Although not common, there are the all-too-true horror stories about the interviewee who is completely unable to answer a freebie like "What courses did you take last semester?" The reason? He was so prepared to perform on a certain level mentally, that when he was asked a straightforward question that had a simple, fact-based answer, his mind sputtered and stalled.

Regardless of the reason, there is a solution to the "in-flight" panic response. As simple as it sounds, the secret is *honesty*. Honesty can extract you gracefully from the toughest of situations. When you are stumped for any reason, do the following: Take a deep breath (this does not have to be dramatic), repeat the question to yourself, and respond with the simple truth. That means admitting when you don't know an answer and admitting when you were wrong.

We are not saying that you won't stutter, or blush, or say "um. . ." more than once. But if you are sincerely dedicated to becoming a doctor, your sincerity and dedication will be obvious to the point that even the most awkward answer will not undermine the overall impression you make.

Notes About Etiquette

First of all, be on time. If you are traveling a great distance, you would be better off arriving the night before your interview. Ask the school about travel arrangements. Some may allow you to stay in the dorms or may have programs in which current medical students offer overnight accommodations in their apartments or houses to applicants traveling for the interview.

If you aren't normally too concerned with personal hygiene and dress, make your interview day an exception. Your appearance should be clean and professional. Most applicants (both male and female) wear suits. If you don't have a suit, try to pull together the most professional attire that you own.

Do not bring food or drink into the interview and do not chew gum. If you smoke, try not to go into the interview smelling like a cigarette. Try not to fidget, nervously shake your legs or feet, tap your fingers or pens, or yawn. The gist here is to be respectful, focused, and attentive. Just take it slow, breathe, and calmly offer your responses.

Remember to write down the name (and proper spelling) of your interviewers. These will be necessary when writing a thank-you note to each interviewer after he or she has met with you. This goes for student interviewers as well. Try to get the notes in the mail as soon as possible after your interview. A brief "thank you" is not only considered polite, it may help them remember you. And in that case, you want their memory triggered before any decisions regarding your future are made.

Common Interview Questions

Highlights

- Most interview questions stem from a handful of basic categories—knowing how you would answer questions in each of these general categories will help prepare you for the interview.
- Know what points you want to make about yourself and use open-ended questions to communicate these points.
- Prepare to speak about any experience, activity, issue, etc. that you included in your essay or elsewhere in your application.
- Knowing your application well and contemplating responses for each of the questions contained in this section will prepare you for the interview.

Ninety percent of unsuccessful interviews are a result of one of two common mistakes made by interviewees. One is being underprepared to answer a specific question; the other is being overprepared. Underpreparation results from the misconception that because it is not possible to predict with accuracy the specific questions that will be asked, it is impossible and/or inefficient to practice answers. The telltale signs of this mistake are meandering, disorganized replies to open-ended questions, contradictions, and redundancies.

The second pitfall, that of overpreparedness, results when good intention is combined with poor strategy. People who make this mistake are easily stumped by unusual questions and may give stilted and overrehearsed answers to more common questions. They might appear to be stiff and nervous, and can even come across as bad listeners, since their answers (though well organized and pointed) do not consistently address the question that was asked. Also, their ability to adapt easily to different interviewers and interview styles is inhibited, making it difficult for them to establish rapport.

This chapter will present a method of preparation that will help you avoid both of these pitfalls. The method stresses both preparedness and flexibility. It takes into account the fact that you can neither predict specific questions nor rely on individually prepared answers.

What we will help you do is prepare generally for the specific. This method of preparation takes advantage of the fact that each of the thousands of possible questions that might be asked is derived from one of a handful of basic categories. We will introduce these general categories and list examples of the specific questions that comprise each. Then we suggest strategies for responding to each type of question.

Your job is this: For each category introduced, arm yourself with at least three points you would like to communicate about yourself and think of one or two specific details to support each. This will allow you to create a targeted, comprehensive set of answers to most of the questions you will be asked. With practice, you will be able to actively use the interviewer's questions (whatever they may be) to communicate the points you wish to make. This puts the control back into your hands, which should also help ease preinterview jitters.

Questions Interviewers Will Ask You

Interviewers are constantly coming up with new and creative questions to ask but no matter how different the question appears to be, it almost always falls into one of the following categories. These categories represent the basics of what the interviewer wants to know about you. If you prepare yourself to speak succinctly in each area, and learn to recognize each question for what it is, you are less likely to be caught off guard by a quirky or unusual query. The categories appear below with examples of some specific questions for each.

Questions from Your Application or Essay

- What compelled you to run the marathon? (or any similar activity you've mentioned)
- Why did you choose that particular research topic?
- How do you stay so focused given your family situation?
- Why did you not write a senior honors thesis?
- Why did you get involved with HIV/AIDS volunteering? (or any similar position mentioned)
- What do you think about "Crime and Punishment" (applicant mentioned Dostoyevsky in his essay)

- Why was the verbal reasoning section of your MCAT low? Do you anticipate this being a problem in medical school?

- Do you think you will be able to compete on the same level as students who speak English as a first language?

- How do you think a degree in Art History has prepared you for medical school?

In some cases, you may have "closed-file" interviews. These are more common with student interviewers. However, most interviewers will have your file in hand and will almost always ask you something triggered directly from your application or your essay. They may ask you to explain weaknesses in your application. They will commonly ask you about interests, issues, and experiences that you wrote about in your essay. Since you are the one who brought it to their attention in the first place, an inability to discuss it would be considered very weak.

Open-Ended Questions

- Who are you?

- Why medical school?

- How would a friend describe you?

- Why do you want to be a doctor?

- How are you unique?

- List three things you want me to know about you.

- What are your strengths and weaknesses?

- Why should we accept you?

- Tell me about yourself.

Open-ended questions are the easiest. There is absolutely no excuse for not taking full advantage of these. First, they are obvious; they are exactly what you should have asked yourself when you first decided to go to medical school. Also, they offer you the chance to openly sell yourself. This is where you should communicate the top three points you would like to make. Preparing specific, focused answers for each of the above questions will also go a long way toward helping you to answer all of the sample questions that follow, no matter what category they are from.

Questions About Your Motivation/Sincerity

- What other careers have you explored?

- Do you feel that you have a realistic view of medical school?

- Do you understand what the life of a doctor entails?

- What will you do if you don't get into medical school?

- Why do you want to attend this school?
- Why do you want to work with sick people?
- Is this school your top choice?
- Where else have you applied?
- Would you consider a foreign medical school?
- Where do you see yourself in 10/20/30 years?
- What do you want to specialize in?
- What do you hope to get out of medicine?
- Do you have any concerns about this school?
- Do you have any ideas about your residency?
- Have you considered the advantages/disadvantages of living in this area?

These questions probe exactly how much you want to practice medicine. The committee wants to understand the thought you have put into your decision. If you have indicated elsewhere in your application that you come from a family of physicians, then they want reassurance that you're not under family pressure. They also need to know that you understand the difficult journey of studying and practicing medicine, and that your knowledge of a doctor's life is not limited to what you have seen on television. Lastly, they want to know that you are sincere in wanting their specific program. If another school is your top choice, be honest. But also be prepared with the reasons that you applied to their school—and it should be more compelling than saying they were your "backup." One tip here is to review the reasons for your motivation that you gave in your essay. The interviewer will probably have read it recently and if your answers don't correspond, it will make the interviewer doubt one or the other—and you.

When answering any one of these questions, start and end with a reiteration of your desire to 1) become a doctor, and 2) attend their school. Emphasize too that you know what your decision entails. Your points should explain why your unique experience makes medical school the right choice. For example: Are you more interested in the science/research side of medicine, or in helping people? If it's the first, you should have a strong research and science background. If it's the latter, back it up with volunteer experience or other kinds of community involvement. Most will stress both sides, which is fine, as long as you can provide solid evidence.

Questions About Your Qualifications and Experience

- What work experience have you had?
- What health-care experience have you had?

- Tell me about your research experience.

- How have you prepared yourself for a career in medicine?

- What clinical/hospital experience have you had?

- What work experience do you wish you had?

- How have you contributed to your community?

- Tell me about a time you have helped someone.

- What volunteer experience have you had?

- What's your toughest subject?

This is pretty straightforward, and easy to prepare for. Just be ready to talk about any experience that you have mentioned in your application. If you feel that you are weak in clinical experience or research, then: 1) say so with regret and explain if there is a good reason, and 2) talk about indirect experience instead (such as the time you set your sister's wrist on a hiking trip or the hours spent tutoring English to adult immigrants). Emphasize your motivation through your experience.

Questions About Your Knowledge of the Medical Field

- What do you see as the biggest challenge facing the field of medicine today?

- Demonstrate your understanding of HMOs, PPOs, and third-party providers.

- Are you aware of the upcoming surplus of doctors? How do you feel about it?

- How do you feel about the debate over the hours residents are forced to work?

- How would you advise patients who are interested in visiting an acupuncturist or chiropractor?

- What do you think about medical advice being available on the Web?

- Express your opinions on:

  - genetic engineering

  - the future of technology in medicine

  - government health-care issues

  - the high cost of health care

  - doctors' salaries

  - hospice care

  - alternative medicine

  - the role of spirituality in healing

This category is often the most daunting for applicants. You might feel that you are being given an oral exam, and on one level you are. The admissions committee wants to see that you are familiar with current events. This is another way to test your sincerity and dedication, and it shows an intellectual curiosity and ability. It is important that the interviewer knows you want to help people, but medicine is as much science as healing and both facets need to be explored.

Questions About Your Personality and Background

- Tell me about a significant event in your life and how it shaped you.
- Do you have a favorite book/class/professor?
- Who do you not get along with and why?
- Which of your qualities would you want to pass down to your children?
- What about yourself would you change if you could?
- What three material objects are most important to you?
- What people have influenced you and how?
- Do you have any heroes?
- How do you handle stress?
- Give me an example of a time you contributed to a group effort.
- Tell me about a cross-cultural experience you have had.
- What do you do in your free time?
- What are your hobbies?
- What is your number one accomplishment?

In some ways these will be easy questions for you. You have had practice with them; they have probably been asked in just about every interview experience you have ever had. These questions about yourself are on more of a superficial level (the more personal questions are discussed below). But talking about yourself—even in response to the lighter questions—can be nerve-wracking when you are being judged on your responses. As always, the answer is to prepare, be yourself, and relax.

Questions About Your Ethics/Character

- Would you work in an AIDS clinic?
- Would you prescribe birth control pills to a minor without parental consent?
- Have you ever cheated or helped a friend cheat?
- How will you deal with know-it-all patients?

- Give your opinions on:
  - genetic engineering
  - abortion
  - euthanasia
  - providing clean needles to addicts
  - supplying condoms to schools
  - animal research

These questions are a subset of questions about the medical field as well as questions about your personality, and subsequently among the toughest to answer. If you are ready for them, though, you will be able to breeze through where others stumble. There are two things that should be of comfort to you: 1) There is a fairly limited number of these "hot" issues so you can be completely ready for most of them, and 2) interviewers won't judge you based on your opinion, even if they disagree, but rather on the thoughtfulness with which you have answered. For this category in particular, preparation is everything.

Personal/Illegal Questions

- Has anyone close to you been seriously ill or died?
- Have you ever been ill or injured?
- What is your relationship with your family like?
- What is more important to you than anything else?
- Are you married/do you have children?
- Do you plan to have children in the future?
- How will you juggle a medical career with a family?
- How important is family to you?
- How do you plan to pay for medical school?

This category is different from the rest. The common thread through these questions is the reluctance of interviewees to answer them, either because they are personal, inappropriate, irrelevant, or illegal. Your first reaction to one of these questions might be embarrassment, discomfort, or annoyance. You might be compelled to refuse an answer, or point out the inappropriateness of the question based on your gender/race, and so on. Our advice is to accept the situation gracefully and answer the question briefly and as straightforwardly as possible. Take into account that the interviewer might be inexperienced, or even testing your ability to tactfully deal with an uncomfortable situation.

Rough Spots

There seem to be more horror stories circulating around the medical school interview than around any other type of interview. The stories end with the interviewees breaking down and crying on the interviewer's shoulder, or freezing up and failing to answer even the simplest of questions. Their propagation is partially due to the fact that medical school is one of the only graduate level schools that, in most cases, requires an interview. At this level of academic rigor, the interview seems even more difficult because most have only the undergraduate interview for comparison, where the interviewers are often more focused on recruiting you than evaluating you. Although it is true that medical school interviews are naturally more harrowing than undergraduate interviews, most of the stories you hear are probably exaggerations. Real disasters rarely happen. Still, there is a lesson to be learned from them: You must prepare yourself to ride gracefully through potential rough spots.

Rough spots can occur when interviewers have little or no experience. They might not know how to prompt you with questions or keep the conversation flowing, and uncomfortable silences might ensue. Or they might be nervous themselves and end up doing most of the talking themselves.

Conversely, you might get an interviewer with too much experience. Perhaps the interviewer has an attitude or seems to want to quiz you on esoteric subjects or prod you for your opinions on touchy medical issues. The interviewer might even ask inappropriate questions about your personal life to see how you respond. A woman, for example, might be asked how she plans to fit her busy schedule into married life, or whether (and how soon) she plans to have children.

Fortunately, these types are rare and you need only remember to remain calm. A level head will help you gracefully admit to not knowing an answer. A sense of humor will help you keep from getting upset. A relaxed attitude will help keep the conversation going when the interviewer fails to do his or her part. In all of these cases, staying focused and relaxed will help you keep your perspective. As long as you don't run screaming from the interviewer's office, it's probably not as bad as you think.

Questions You Can Ask Interviewers

One question you can count on being asked in every interview is: "Do you have any questions?" There is a correct answer to this question. It is unequivocally "Yes!" Your questions should be as well planned and as revealing as an answer to any other question they have asked. Use your questions to show that you have done your research. Because the questions should be specific to you, we advise that you come up with your own personal questions and don't rely on the suggestions that we provide below. Just keep two points in mind and any question will do:

1. Don't ask anything that can be easily researched.
2. Don't ask objective questions twice of different interviewers at the same school as they may compare notes later.

Questions for the Faculty Interviewer

- How much of the curriculum will be lecture time and how much will be small group sessions?
- Where and what are typical alumni doing now?
- Do alumni tend to stay in the area after graduation?
- What are the school's weaknesses?
- What are the school's strengths?
- When do students have their first contact with patients?

Questions for the Student Interviewer

- How would you rate the faculty here?
- In your opinion, do the students like it here?
- What sort of clinical/research opportunities are available?
- What is a typical day like for a first-year student?
- What makes your school unique?
- What do you like about this school?
- How would you describe the students here?

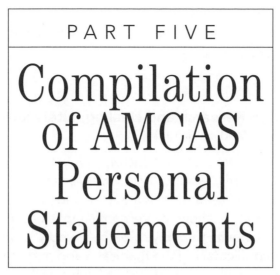

PART FIVE

Compilation of AMCAS Personal Statements

The upcoming pages contain authentic AMCAS personal statements. The essays are not samples; they are real essays written by candidates who were accepted into the top medical schools in the United States. The school where each candidate was accepted is listed before each essay, along with some tags to help you quickly identify the essays that will be most relevant to you. Students' comments can be found under some of the essays revealing such facts as the amount of time it took them to write their statement and how much weight they thought the statement had in their overall application. In addition, you will find comments by the authors of this book on the strengths of each essay and, with the exception of a few that left no room for improvement, we've also provided our opinion on how each could have been made even stronger.

All mistakes, typos, grammar, and spelling errors found in the original essays have been preserved. Despite these occasional surface errors, the essays were written by some of the most qualified applicants in the world and the quality of them is, on the whole, outstanding. Do not let this intimidate you. Use them as a learning tool and as a source of inspiration.

Plagiarizing from these or any essays is illegal. Because IvyEssays works with admissions officers from schools around the country, the committees are familiar with the essays presented here and will likely know if material you are using has been taken from the examples in this book.

To help you sort quickly through the statements that are most relevant to you, we suggest you use the index at the back of the book that catalogs each essay according to theme, the writer's related experience and background, and the schools to which they were accepted. We hope you enjoy them, and wish you the best of luck in your application process.

ESSAY 1: Bridging Research and Healing, Literature Background
Accepted at: Mayo Medical School

When I think of practicing as a doctor, I am most concerned about the intersection of scientific research and society's capacity to apply it, both in terms of legislation regarding health care and in terms of my ability as a doctor to comprehend how this research applies to my patient's health. Society's inability to apply research soundly is what I consider to be the biggest conflict facing the medical world and our larger society. For a doctor to be well educated and well informed does not automatically result in the best diagnosis in this day and age. The amount of new scientific information that medical research is producing almost daily becomes absolutely staggering, even for the specialist. And the medical establishment is currently under pressure to emphasize general practice, under the title "primary care." How can we expect this new wave of physicians to consistently give the highest quality of care, especially given the difficulty doctors have in correctly interpreting medical research findings? This difficulty was highlighted in a survey Health magazine recently conducted, which showed that only 25% of the doctors could correctly take raw data, or even a statistical analysis of the data, and turn it into a good diagnosis for their patients.

We are currently living in a society still split between the isolated world of scientific research and the much larger world of politicians, legislators, artists, writers, and those who comprise our social services. This split is a particularly dangerous now, given the incredible influence the words "backed by scientific research" confer to advertising, which usually converts into the health trends of our society. Too few people exist whose vocation it is to bridge these two worlds, to bring accurate understanding to the majority of our society, and of these, doctors are the most important. In 1964, the scientist and philosopher C. P. Snow wrote about the split between these two cultures, which he called the scientific and the literary, saying: "It is dangerous to have two cultures which can't or don't communicate. In a time when science is determining much of our destiny, that is, whether we live or die, it is dangerous in the most practical terms. Scientists can give bad advice and decision-makers can't know whether it is good or bad." How can we solve this conundrum facing the medical establishment? C. P. Snow advised an overhaul in the way the Western world educates its children, in which young people would study the sciences as rigorously as they studied the humanities, and in the American liberal arts college system, he saw his idea come to fruition.

I am a product of this system, having learned science, as well as literature, from the first day in my private school kindergarten class. In fact, my dual love of literature and science caused me inner conflict when, in high school, I was deciding what I wanted to do with my college studies, and ultimately with my life. I had then, as I do now, a deep passion for literature; however, as becoming a doctor was my highest priority, I wanted to be well-prepared for medical school. I needed to decide how to balance my fascination with scientific problems with my need for artistic expression. My senior year at Wellesley College exemplified my solution to this problem.

During that year, I produced an Honors senior research thesis on William Faulkner that was the culmination of a four-year dream, had two of my fiction short stories published in news magazines at Stanford and the University of California at Los Angeles, performed surgery on rats and designed behavioral tests for rat spatial memory using a Morris Water Maze as part of my neurological research class. My outstanding skill in analyzing literature helped me to understand how to analyze scientific research, as I sifted through multiple papers to discover what theories were relevant to my current research endeavors. In the same manner, I had to uncover for my thesis a sound basis for challenging some of the purveying theories concerning William Faulkner's writings. I found I was using the same pattern of thinking in what are commonly regarded as disciplines that require widely disparate types of thinking, most commonly expressed as "different kinds of people." After years of being unable to explain why I could excel and enjoy both the sciences and the humanities, I finally realized that they both required similar abilities. A balance between the scientific and literary worlds of C. P. Snow was not necessarily required for our society's continued health; instead, what was required was a synthesis of the drive to know and to solve and the drive to create and to express. I found that this balance in thinking was equally necessary to scientific or to liberal arts endeavors, and that the balance that is so necessary for our society's physicians to have, and that C. P. Snow so strongly advocated, was not between two disciplines—science and liberal arts—but between two types of thinking—analytical and creative. I believe that it is my strength in both of these areas, as shown by my research interests coupled with a degree in the humanities, that makes me so well suited to be a physician. I know that in medicine, I can excel as one of those bridges between the science that is so critical to our health and those who we are devoted to healing.

Strengths

The essay is well written and well structured. The author has two main themes (the practical application of scientific research and the applicant's passion for both literature and science) and she molds them together into a cohesive essay where each topic is relevant to her pursuit of a career in medicine. She demonstrates intelligence and a motivation to study medicine through her discussion of both topics. She weaves in achievements, which are evidence of her ability to succeed, through the experiences that she shares as an undergraduate.

Weaknesses

The applicant has several long sentences that would be easier to digest if she broke them down into two or more shorter sentences or if she had been able to express the same thoughts in fewer words.

ESSAY 2: Mother's Illness; West Point Graduate; Clinical Experience in General Surgery

Accepted at: University of Pennsylvania School of Medicine; Cornell University Medical College; Harvard Medical School; Tufts University School of Medicine; University of Cincinnati College of Medicine; Georgetown University School of Medicine; Mount Sinai School of Medicine, CUNY

My desire to become a doctor traces back to my childhood memories. Vividly, I remember my mother's tragic experience. I was only six years old when she underwent a tracheostomoy. The days following the surgical procedure were incredibly frustrating. Not only was she confined to her bed, but she was unable to speak to me as well. I felt so helpless, and all I wanted was for her to be well again.

The most prominent memories I have of my mother's experience are seldomly leaving her side and helping her to clean and change her tube. Because of this, everyone felt I was the most concerned about her. My family kept telling me I would be a great doctor some day. That idea stuck with me, and now, through my own volition, I still want to become a physician.

I came to West Point knowing that if I wanted to fulfill my dream of becoming a physician, I would have to distinguish myself. People warned me that West Point is probably not the best undergraduate institution for someone with a desire to become a physician, since only 2 percent of the Academy graduates are allowed to attend medical school. Everything I have done here has been geared toward preparing myself for medical school and insuring that I would be one of the 2 percent.

I began my undergraduate education by taking organic chemistry as a freshman, again against the advice of many people. I knew I would be successful in this 300-level course, and I was. The summer before my junior year, I spent three weeks at Walter Reed Medical Center in Washington, DC to gain clinical experience. At Walter Reed the surgeons treated me as if I was a third-year medical student. I was given unlimited access to the operating rooms and was encouraged to follow the progress of several patients. Futhermore, when I rotated through general surgery, I was allowed to scrub in and be an integral member of the surgical team on four cases. The program was such an enjoyable and informative experience that I participated in it again the summer before my senior year in lieu of taking vacation.

As it has turned out, the people who warned me against West Point as a premedical institution were grossly mistaken. Very few institutions demand the same time and stress management that West Point has forced me to learn. These skills will prove to be invaluable to me not only as a medical student but as a doctor as well. In addition to West Point's prestigious academic program, it is renowned as the greatest leadership institution in the world. This latter aspect of the Academy has further developed my interpersonal and leadership skills, again two skills that will be most useful to me as a student and doctor.

The Military Academy develops a certain type of person—a well-rounded leader who is capable of accomplishing anything. I took a risk by coming to West Point—the risk of failing to distinguish myself among an elite group of people, thereby postponing my medical education for at least five years. But I succeeded in my risk, and I will be one of the proud 2 percent in my class who is allowed to attend medical school.

Student Comments

I feel this is a very generic medical school personal statement, but I think that overall, the ideas that come across were very important in getting me into medical school. It's from the heart (which is what admissions committees want to see) and it lets the reader get to know me (through college). Because of time commitments (as all premeds have), I only allowed myself to put this essay together in two nights. The first night I wrote the rough draft, and I proofread it the next. No other persons read the essay before I submitted it (in retrospect, not a good idea).

As a current member of the admissions committee at Harvard and a premedical advisor at Harvard College, I realize that the personal statement is the only way that an admissions committee member can get to know an applicant and therefore, the essay should be written and rewritten, read and proofread, countless times! I clearly did not put the time into this essay that I should have, and I am fortunate that the rest of my application carried enough weight to earn me acceptances.

Strengths

The applicant was able to pull off a standard personal statement in a short period of time that obviously did not hurt his application.

Weaknesses

The essay should have been more personal and interesting. Discussing other people's objections to his decision to attend West Point and taking organic chemistry as a freshman not only led to uninteresting paragraphs, they came across as a bit arrogant. Both are included elsewhere in his application as well. The applicant should have spoken more about his experiences and through them, let his qualifications and achievements speak for themselves.

ESSAY 3: Career Switcher from Marketing Management; Lab Experience; Assistant to Athletic Trainer
Accepted at: Harvard Medical School

I was not in control of my life and I was miserable. Forced by my parents' unwillingness to pay for my education, I worked as a branch manager for a marketing corporation. From April to September, I spent twelve to fourteen hours at work each day, doing everything possible to make enough money to return to school the following year. Amid the hard work, I lost track of who I was and what I wanted in life. I lost touch with my friends and the people that I cared about.

In spite of this, the experience was worthwhile. As a manager in charge of 46 people, I learned valuable skills of communication and personal interaction which related to my goal of working in the medical profession. Everyday, I had the opportunity to interview several new people, to talk to them, and get to know a little about them. In addition, through functions in and out of the office, I became very close with the core of my sales force. Not only did I teach them how to sell our product, but I listened to their personal problems and gave them advice. As a result, I had the pleasure of receiving a letter from one of my salespersons at the end of the summer thanking me for the skills that she had learned and the self-confidence that she had gained.

Later that year, however, I decided to begin to regain control of my life. Although I realized that it would increase financial pressures, I chose to stop working for the marketing corporation and prepare more directly for a career in medicine. I accepted a job in a laboratory at the University of Pennsylvania School of Medicine in order to broaden my experience and ensure that I was choosing the right profession.

In high school, I had experience dealing directly with patients. I assisted the athletic trainer, taping players, treating injuries, and making diagnoses. The experience was enjoyable because I learned a great deal about sports medicine, including anatomy and muscle function. It also showed me the importance of teamwork in medicine. Having been an athlete, I recognized the power of teamwork on the field. Yet, I had been unaware of the cooperation needed in the training room. The most worthwhile aspect of the experience, however, was the trust and respect that the players showed towards me. After I became comfortable working by myself, I could sense that they felt secure when I treated them.

Research was new to me, yet I was impressed by the intellectual challenges that it presented. I appreciated the systematic approach and planning that were required to solve problems and direct research. I liked the attention to detail that was needed to be successful. I enjoyed the atmosphere of the laboratory and the cooperative spirit of the researchers. Most of all, however, I was attracted by the idea that I could have impact on many lives by conducting research.

The research experience that I have had, combined with my sister's recent cancer diagnosis and therapy, changed my view on my future in medicine. Previously, I had planned to work only in the clinic, so that I could have personal contact with patients. Now, I also feel a responsibility to contribute to the advancement of medical science. I intend to perform research so that others may avoid hardships like the one that my sister has undergone during the past year. Focused on my career goal, I have retaken control of my life. I have decided what I want to do and who I want to be. I have found a career that will balance my intellectual curiosity with my longing for personal interaction. I have found a career that will engage my interests and will be fulfilling for me.

Strengths

The essay has an intriguing introduction. From the first sentence, the reader gets the sense that this essay is going to be personal and is interested in reading more. The first couple of paragraphs that discuss the applicant's career in marketing are effective for two reasons. First, his hard-working and determined nature is revealed in the fact that he got a real job to pay for his own education. Second, he manages to make his brief career in marketing relevant by describing how it motivated him to make further advances toward a career in medicine.

Weaknesses

The essay is underdeveloped. It fails to be as personal as it promised to be in the beginning. The experiences that are relayed do not explain why a career in medicine is the applicant's ultimate goal. The research that was briefly mentioned was not described with any level of detail. Finally, the conclusion is made up of too many bold statements that are not evidenced by the applicant's experiences.

ESSAY 4: Motivated since Childhood; Nursing Home Volunteer; Peer Counselor; ADD Tutor; Research Experience in Genetics and Rheumatology
Accepted at: Harvard Medical School

"I love the way he makes me laugh." "She's so cute when she crinkles her nose." "He's the most intelligent person I know." These sentiments are often expressed to support the decision to marry. However, they undoubtedly do not reflect the criteria employed to choose a spouse. Proper questioning can evoke the genuine reason. "It is a feeling from my heart. I know that only with this person will I feel complete." It is in the same almost ineffable way that I passionately desire to be a physician. The commitment is much akin to marrying. Various experiences have shaped my conviction. With no less consideration than I would exercise regarding a marriage, have I arrived at my decision.

I first recognized my inclination towards medicine many years ago, when my grandmother sliced her finger preparing dinner. Discovering that she owned no "band-aids," I flushed with excitement from being in a position to care for her. I hurriedly concocted an original bandage from scotch tape and cotton, and presented it to her. My high school volunteer work at a local nursing home reminded me of this incident. It also reawakened my desire to understand more about the causes of disease. I spent much time reading and conversing with the elderly residents in the home. While my capacity to affect them greatly gratified me, my inability to medically help them frustrated me. I promised myself I would learn as much as possible so I could help more in the future.

My involvement in tutoring and peer counseling have also reinforced my desire to practice medicine as well as helped to cultivate my communication skills. Many members of my family suffer from Attention Deficit Disorder. Maturing in this environment motivated and prepared me to knowledgeably aid others with the condition. I have devoted many hours to tutoring ADD-diagnosed children. This activity has challenged me to become proficient at explaining ideas with easily graspable examples. I have also realized that encouragement is almost as important as the actual knowledge imparted. As a peer counselor, I am available as resource or listener for students. Outside of class, an acquaintance once sought my help in solving a personal problem. I felt honored when he chose to confide in me because he affirmed my ability to empathize and listen without prejudice.

As an undergraduate, I have desired to augment my studies with research. I initially performed genetic experiments with Drosophila melanogaster. Last semester, I began studying the genes and proteins used by Escherichia coli to catabolize the disaccharide chitobiose. Chitobiose is derived from chitin, the second most abundant polysaccharide in nature. This endeavor has complemented the biochemistry coursework that I enjoyed immensely, by providing practical applications for it. Daily, I utilize the invaluable techniques of molecular cloning, PCR, and gel electrophoresis. As a Howard Hughes Summer Research Fellow, I am continuing this research. I relish the opportunity to conduct laboratory investigations that will be pivotal to my comprehension of future medical breakthroughs.

Working in conjunction with a rheumatologist at Johns Hopkins School of Medicine last summer solidified my passion for clinical medicine. I investigated pregnancy complications and possible hormone predictors of preterm delivery in lupus patients. The study began with a review of the primary literature regarding corticotropin-releasing hormone and prolactin and a presentation to the Rheumatology Grand Rounds. Additionally, I observed patient visits to the outpatient clinic and hospital. Through the summer and following semester, I continued to speak with patients, review their medical charts, and complete a vast database of medical histories and hormone levels. I witnessed the realities of being a doctor: The frustration of patient non-compliance, the alarming restrictions imposed by insurance companies, and the inherent limitations of modern medicine for treating certain ailments. Nevertheless, I also experienced the most rewarding moments, such as the recovery of patients believing themselves to be dying. I especially enjoyed my contact with the patients and am eager to establish a strong rapport with patients of my own.

The challenges inherent in medicine entice me to become a physician. After sampling related activities, I can confidently assert that I love clinical medicine. As Emerson once said, "People wish to be settled; only as far as they are unsettled is there any hope for them." The medical field never stagnates. As a physician, I will be privy to the fantastic and incessant advances occurring in medicine. Only this constant influx of knowledge will satisfy my insatiable desire to comprehend the human body and its relation to the world. It will inspire me to continue learning and contributing to improving the health of others. Just as a marriage retains its vibrancy when the partners actively partake in new pursuits, by its nature, medicine has an invigorating quality that will forever engage me.

Strengths

This is a strong essay. It has a unique introduction that is tied nicely to the conclusion. The applicant demonstrates her commitment to the study of medicine through almost every experience that she relates. She discusses her research with the perfect amount of detail—enough to satisfy the committee's interest without turning the essay into a research paper.

Weaknesses

The second paragraph tells two separate stories. It should have been broken down into two separate paragraphs.

ESSAY 5: Motivated since Childhood; Family of Physicians; High School Hospital Volunteer; High School Student Council; Resident Advisor; Research Experience in Cloning and Gene Therapy
Accepted at: Harvard Medical School

Dr. Lewis Thomas described medicine as "The Youngest Science" because insightful discoveries in basic research have led to revolutionary innovations in clinical therapy that have improved the quality of life. We are in an the midst of an exciting era in which our knowledge about the molecular aspects of medicine is growing each day. I feel that the medical profession uniquely integrates my passion for science with my desire to work with others. Medicine is boundless; like no other profession, it wholly captures my intellectual ideals and humanistic values.

I have been curious about medicine since childhood. To learn about the profession, I would pose questions to the physicians in my own family. Eager to gain hands on experience, I volunteered in high school at the St. Joseph's Hospital in [hometown]. I had the opportunity to escort patients from one area of the hospital to another prior to diagnostic tests or treatments. Through interactions with many patients, I discovered the therapeutic and comforting effects of an encouraging smile and a friendly conversation. From observing patients with simple correctable problems, such as a hernia, to those with chronic problems, such as rheumatoid arthritis, I gained an understanding for a physician's daily challenges. Each patient presented a complex array of symptoms that required specialized attention. In order for a physician to help a patient cope with an illness, it was important for him to consider the patient's emotional needs. Especially in stressful situations, I appreciated how the reassuring confidence and warmth, conveyed through a physician's bedside manner, gradually transformed a patient's immediate fears into strength and hope.

Medicine offers diverse opportunities to interact with others. In the past, I have found service-oriented activities to be particularly rewarding. In high school, I felt that I could most effectively contribute to my local community by participating in student government. As Student Council President, I interacted with individuals with a variety of personalities to ensure that my peers had the opportunity to express their ideas and opinions freely. At [name] University, I discovered that the most vital component of campus life was living in the residence hall. Therefore, after my freshman year, I decided to become a Resident Advisor (RA). One of my personal goals was to encourage each resident to take full advantage of our unique living situation. As a diverse community, we had many experiences to share with each other. I enjoyed organizing activities such as discussions, educational programs, and study breaks that helped form an interactive and supportive community. For the past two years, some of my most rewarding experiences have emerged from my dynamic role as a peer counselor and resource figure. One of the most challenging situations that I encountered was when our floor custodian informed me about the packaged bags of regurgitated food that he found in the women's bathroom over several weeks. By consulting fellow staff members and recruiting the help of health professionals, my co-RA and I organized educational programs about eating disorders to address this sensitive situation. Fortunately, there were no further occurrences. By helping my peers cope with the stresses of college life as an RA, I not only gained valuable interpersonal skills, but also formed lasting friendships.

Another interest that I have explored is my fascination with the creative and unpredictable diversity of living organisms. With a fervent interest in biology, I joined the genetics laboratory of Dr. X. in my freshman year. After learning about the biology of the ciliated protozoan, Tetrahymena thermophila, I focused my efforts on understanding the mechanism of strain-specific, age-dependent micronuclear degradation. With the support of the Howard Hughes Scholar Program for Undergraduates, I cloned transposon-like elements in Tetrahymena that may cause chromosomal rearrangements associated with age-dependent micronuclear degradation. The multitude of puzzles that I encountered in the laboratory challenged my creativity and fostered intellectual development that I could not attain in a classroom. By critically analyzing experimental obstacles, I gained invaluable problem solving skills. In my senior year, I will further investigate this intriguing model of aging as part of my honors thesis.

Because my research experience has added a unique dimension to my education, I feel that it is important to support the research interests of others. As an executive board member of the [name] Undergraduate Research Board, I have assisted students in finding faculty members with similar research interests. This past year, I took part in organizing a forum for students to present their research findings to the Cornell community.

This summer, I have engaged in an internship that has enhanced my understanding of the relationship between basic research and medicine. By working with Dr. [name] at the Memorial Sloan-Kettering Cancer Center, I discovered the excitement that surrounds the emerging science and technology that will lead to future innovations in medicine. A long term goal of Dr. [name]'s laboratory is to develop retroviral-mediated gene therapy for patients with chronic hemolytic anemia due to a severe deficiency of glucose-6-phosphate dehydrogenase (G6PD). I tested the efficiency of replication-defective retroviral vectors that are capable of transferring the human G6PD gene to cells in vitro. The existence of inherited diseases such as severe G6PD deficiency, cystic fibrosis, adenosine deaminase deficiency, and others that are clinically manageable, but incurable, presents a unique problem to the medical community. Ideally, I wish to be involved in both the traditional primary care of these patients and investigative research that may lead to more effective therapy.

I aspire to become a physician because to me, it is the world's most vibrant and rewarding profession. The practice of medicine offers a daily sense of fulfillment that is rare. Basic and clinical research enhances our understanding of disease and provides us with the tools to improve the lives of many. As a lifelong commitment to society, the medical profession most completely encompasses my career goals and moral values.

Strengths

This is a comprehensive essay that gives the reader a sense of who the applicant is and confirms that she has been motivated to pursue a career in medicine for a long time. Through her experiences, she demonstrates that she is well rounded and competent.

Weaknesses

The essay is too long and the applicant focuses too much on her high school experiences. The volunteer experience is fine as it demonstrates an early interest in medicine. However, she should not have transitioned to her experience as student government president because, at that point, she included more high school experience than the admissions committee cares to hear. The majority of experiences should be timeless (in that they reveal an applicant's character or motivations) or they should be more recent.

ESSAY 6: Musician/Drummer; Religious Catholic; Science and Math Tutor; Cancer Research Experience
Accepted at: Harvard Medical School

The beating of an African healing drum resonates throughout all corners of the Catholic church during the weekly five o'clock student mass. As I progressively increase the tempo and intensity of the resounding Guaguanca polyrhythm that I am playing, the congregation begins to sway back and forth to the beat. Soon the members start clapping in unison on the quarter notes. By the end of the hymn, they are dancing in place and singing along in high spirits. The mass is truly a celebration.

While a drumming performance in church may appear a little unorthodox, the concept of rhythm has never seemed very offbeat to me. Music has always been a motivating passion in my life. My desire to play percussion was evident as early as third grade, when I would tap my pencil on the top of my classroom desk and kick the chair in front to simulate a bass drum. Rhythm seemed so fundamental to me. Besides being bombarded with it through popular pop music, I could hear it in every tick of the clock, each person's gait, my own heartbeat. I longed to master it— to be able to manipulate it, incorporate it into my own being, and then finally convey it to others. I began drum lessons. After seven years of basic mechanical training, I developed my own style. Talent shows, parties, dances, even religious ceremonies became forums for my expression. I joined a band in high school which became the ticket to a performance in Disneyworld. As a Christian Service project, my rock band performed at various inner-city grammar schools, hospitals, and nursing homes. In college, my main band became known as Harvard's newest sensation. Soon we found ourselves performing in various clubs, parties, and school-sponsored concerts, and our recording culminated in the production of a CD. I even began to convey my knowledge to a beginner, and had the pleasure of watching him grow in much the same manner as I had. The musical frontier seemed limitless.

Concurrently, my passion for science began to crystallize. I had always participated in the annual school science fairs and after-school science-related activities, but it was not until high school that I really began to appreciate my penchant for scientific reasoning. After learning the fundamental concepts, I sought any opportunity to demonstrate them in a creative manner. Everything was a puzzle. In an extracurricular high school program, I constructed a Bausch & Lomb award-winning contraption which integrated numerous laws of physics. I took this a step further when I began to realize that I could demonstrate my love for science in a way that could benefit others. I volunteered full-time in the emergency room of a local hospital during the last trimester of senior year. It was here that I caught my first glimpse of hands-on medicine. During the next few years, I tutored high school students in science and math. In addition to the personal satisfaction obtained from observing their progress, this provided an excellent opportunity to hone my communication and teaching skills. Last summer, I worked in a cancer research laboratory in Memorial Sloan-Kettering Hospital, attempting to isolate a gene that encoded for limb development in Drosophila. By September, our team had fully mapped and cloned Chip and was preparing for publication. Senior thesis work on comparative avian, reptilian, and mammalian bone morphology also enabled me to integrate rudimentary mechanics and personal interaction with professors and fellow peers.

It has become clear that the most attractive features to me in the diverse fields of science and music are one and the same. Music is a creative art form that conveys feelings and emotions in a manner unlike any other form of expression. It is, in a sense, a fascinating language with universal appeal. Science is both an art form and an exercise in methodology. Part of its nature is strictly mechanistic, yet its application is also an exercise in expression and communication. I certainly appreciate the beauty and elegance of the underlying principles in both disciplines. However, it is the expression of these ideas and subsequent communication to others that inspires me the most. My devotion to science and music has had a complimentary effect that has served both to enhance my method of thinking and to fulfill my yearning to communicate. I hope to continue to relate with others in the field of medicine, where creative application of science and keen expression is essential. I know that my concept of the rhythm of life will help keep me grounded in the fundamentals as I strive to convey and apply my knowledge and gifts to others.

Strengths

This is a fantastic essay. It is very well written, beginning with an interesting discussion of the applicant's passion for music. This discussion is effectively woven into a satisfying conclusion. The discussion of music is tied to the applicant's second theme, his passion for science. His motivations are clear and believable. His talent makes him unique. His writing is so solid and seemingly effortless that his intelligence and ability to communicate are unquestioned. The essay is a pleasure to read and will help the applicant stand out from the crowd.

Weaknesses

None.

ESSAY 7: Liberal Arts/Theater Background; Lab Experience in Reproductive Ecology; Teaching Assistant; Clinical Research Experience and Women's Clinic Volunteer

Admitted at: University of Pennsylvania School of Medicine; Harvard Medical School; Tufts University School of Medicine

It was opening night. I was about to walk on stage as Ruth in *The Pirates of Penzance*. Any sane actor would be singing scales, or meditating, or reviewing dialogue. I was spitting into a test tube. Later, I would assay the saliva for cortisol and compare the results with my normal cortisol levels. Discovering what was happening in my body as the curtain prepared to rise was worth the temporary distraction from the pirate king.

"Spit happens," as we say in my lab. Spit happened to me during the summer after my sophomore year in college. I worked in the Reproductive Ecology Laboratory at Harvard University, measuring steroid hormones in saliva by radioimmunoassay. I had never considered myself a science whiz, and I took the job with a little trepidation. I pipetted until my thumb ached and washed an endless stream of glassware, but the end result was something amazing. With those tiny vials of saliva, I could track my menstrual cycle. I could measure my brother's testosterone levels, or my own—which I hadn't even known I had. I realized that I was doing science. I was doing it well and enjoying it. I went on to complete my senior honors thesis on the relationship between cortisol levels and temperament in shy adolescents. In the lab, I discovered the fascination of research and the discipline needed to carry it out.

About the same time spit happened to me, I found myself writing research papers on a consistent set of themes. For my women's history class, I wrote about the turn of the century movement for "twilight sleep" anesthesia in childbirth. For my sophomore tutorial in anthropology, I researched the effects of social support on the duration and complications of labor and delivery. For my sociology class, I investigated the controversy surrounding the Depo Provera contraceptive. My passion for these topics and my interest in science fueled a growing desire to go to medical school. I began taking pre-med classes and continued pursuing these interests, both in and out of the classroom.

At Lutheran General Hospital in Park Ridge, Illinois, I studied patients who had undergone laparoscopic surgery for uterine fibroids and ovarian cysts. While gathering clinical data, reading literature, and observing surgeries, I was amazed by the results of such non-invasive techniques, and had visions of holding the laparoscope myself in a few years. I enjoyed being part of the rhythms of a busy obstetrics and gynecology practice and solidified my desire to be a doctor.

As a volunteer in a women's health clinic in Boston, during my senior year in college, I answered phones and made appointments and referrals. I discovered how much good I could do just by listening and focusing my attention on the person on the phone. That simple act did so much to alleviate a woman's worries and uncertainties. I also learned to treat each patient with fairness and decency, regardless of her circumstances. I know that the things I can accomplish listening with the additional skills of a physician are extraordinary.

Much of my remaining spare time in college was spent working in theater. While president of the Harvard-Radcliffe Gilbert and Sullivan Players, I led a board of fifteen strong-willed, outspoken peers. I made sure each person was heard in discussions and that the group remained focused. As producer of several plays, I was thrilled to watch the curtain rise, knowing I had harnessed the energies and talents of dozens of people to make the show happen. Through my work in theater, I learned to keep my stress levels reasonable and my temper intact while juggling innumerable tasks—usually on very few hours of sleep.

In college, I became one part scientist, one part counselor, and one part leader. My interest in how our bodies work and how we relate to those bodies continues to grow in tandem with my vision of myself as a physician. I know that with the skills I gained in college, from techniques in the laboratory to group leadership in theater production to listening and compassion on the clinic telephone, I am well prepared to enter medical school. And I can't wait to see what it does to my cortisol levels.

Student Comments:

As I recall, it took me between six and eight weeks to write this essay, including time to mail it back and forth to my premed advisor for critiquing. In the original version, I fantasized about being trapped in an elevator with a pregnant woman and delivering her baby while we waited for the repairmen. My advisor felt that scenario was too frivolous and silly sounding, so I changed it to the (true) story that starts this version.

Strengths

This is a very solid and entertaining essay. It has a fantastic introduction because it tells a comical story, makes the applicant immediately likable and interesting, and ties the story to her passion for science all within a few short sentences. She has a witty introduction to the next paragraph, which begins her discussion of research. She describes her research with the perfect amount of detail and is one of the few applicants that is convincingly passionate about it. Her experience in theater helps present her as a well-rounded and unique applicant who can successfully juggle a full and diverse workload. Her wit is once again showcased in her tidy conclusion.

Weaknesses

None.

ESSAY 8: Counselor/Teacher for Refugee Youth Program and Emotionally Disturbed Children's Camp
Accepted at: Columbia University College of Physicians and Surgeons (offered $40,000 scholarship); Cornell University Medical College; Duke University School of Medicine; University of Michigan Medical School (also offered $20,000 scholarship); Harvard Medical School

Roasting marshmallows on chopsticks over a gas grill, I looked back on how much my relationship with M. had deepened over the two years that we had known each other. M., a thirteen-year-old refugee from Vietnam, had been one of my summer students in the Boston Refugee Youth Enrichment (BRYE) program. On this May night, the two of us were going on a camping trip in M.'s backyard. M. was very well-prepared for our adventure: a poster bearing the stern admonition "KEEP AWAY" protected a tent packed with flashlights, pillows, board games, and peanut butter and cheese crackers. These careful arrangements reflected M.'s excitement about the overnight that we were braving together; I shared this excitement, and realized how fortunate I was to be spending this night with my student and close friend.

Certainly, M. would not have been excited at the prospect of spending an overnight together when he entered my class two years earlier. M. had had behavioral problems during past summers in BRYE, and the BRYE program directors placed him in my class because of my experience [at] Camp R., a camp for emotionally disturbed children. Indeed, M.'s behavior was less than exemplary on the first day of BRYE, and I remember feeling daunted by the challenge of fostering respect between us. Yet somehow, between that first crazy day of BRYE Summer and the night of our camping trip two years later, M. and I had moved beyond the guarded relationship of teacher and class troublemaker; we had become very special friends who trusted each other enough to face together the urban wilderness of Dorchester, Massachusetts.

I am not exactly sure how this change occurred; I often find it difficult to identify specific events that have shaped my relationships with M. and others to whom I have grown close through my work with BRYE and Camp R. However, I remember particularly well staying up one night with C., an eight-year-old boy in my bunk at Camp R., after he had been terribly frightened by a nightmare in which spiders were devouring him. I gave C. my high school gym uniform to wear, suggesting that its ugly, bright orange color might deter spiders with their sensitive compound eyes. Then I sat on his bed and guarded him from spiders until he was able to fall asleep again.

More recently this past February, I had the opportunity to celebrate Tet, the Vietnamese New Year, with the family of B., one of my students from last summer. B.'s family had been well off before the Communist government took away all that they owned with the victory of North

Vietnam over the South in 1975. After the father's imprisonment in a re-education camp for his ties to the South Vietnamese military, the family came to the United States. Soon after their arrival, their new home burned down, exacerbating the hardships that they faced in this country. Nevertheless, eating, talking, and laughing with B. and his sisters, mother, father, and grandmother, I was greatly moved by the strength and resilience that had emerged from this family's love for one another, and deeply honored that they were willing to share this important holiday with me.

These relationships that I have had with M., C., B.'s family, and others have been very meaningful because we have established genuine, mutual trust. C. could feel safe in the knowledge that I would stay by his bed as long as he needed, and I treasured his honesty in sharing his feelings with me. B.'s family recognized the sincerity of my respect for them, just as I was comfortable knowing that their affection and respect for me were genuine as well. Such trust, I believe, is the foundation of the relationships I have formed over the past four years, and has fostered a closeness that has impacted my life very deeply. Moreover, the importance of trust in the friendships I have had with others has significantly influenced the expectations, goals and dreams that I have for myself today, including my aspirations for a career in medicine.

My hopes to become a physician were not always motivated by this desire to grow from and give to trusting relationships with others. Since childhood, I have wanted to be a doctor, and it was a sincere fascination with life that first sparked my enthusiasm for medicine. Nothing seemed more amazing to me than the human body, and I thought that I would be fortunate if I could dedicate my life to so challenging and interesting a study. As a child I was eager to understand how the body fends off illness and to explore the fate of food after it is eaten; now I hope to grasp the answers to these and other questions well enough that I can confront successfully many of the challenges that I will face as a doctor.

The people with whom I have shared myself, however, have shown me that being a doctor means more than making a correct diagnosis and applying an appropriate treatment. To me, being a doctor means fostering trust between myself and my patients, so that we can enjoy mutual confidence as we enrich our own lives through shared experiences. It also means establishing trust with my peers. The friendships that I have made with other counselors have been some of the best aspects of my experiences with BRYE and Camp R. Two of my closest friends, T., a year older than I, and S., a year younger, have played especially important roles in my personal growth over the past few years. None of us knew right away the significance that working with Dorchester's Vietnamese refugee community would hold for us. However, through sharing our insights into the challenges, failures, and successes we experienced, as well as our passion for the work we were doing, each of us grew and learned more together than any one of us could have done on our own. Similarly, given the demands of becoming a good doctor, I believe that many of my colleagues will share a passion for medicine akin to S. and T.'s passion for BRYE. I very much hope to be a part of such a community of men and women who, through facing together the challenges and hardships of being physicians, enrich each other's lives just as they enrich the lives of the patients to whom they have dedicated themselves.

Thus, after my experiences over the past four years with BRYE and Camp R., I believe that my commitment to the medical profession will be a commitment, above all else, to the children, women and men whom I serve, as well as to the men and women with whom I serve. Although I realize that I cannot become lifelong friends with everyone I meet, I hope that the comfort we feel in our mutual trust and respect will make some difference in our lives. Indeed, I am sometimes daunted by the difficulty I will inevitably face in encouraging others to place their trust in me as I place my trust in them, for I will not always be able to fulfill the needs of everyone whom I serve. Nevertheless, I am eager to make this commitment, for no experiences in my life have been as happy or gratifying as those that I have shared intimately with others. If, as a doctor, I can continue giving to, learning from, and sharing with others as I have as a counselor and teacher over the past four years, I believe that my life will be a fulfilling one; it is to this end that I hope to dedicate myself. Reminiscing about how M. pulled the browned marshmallow from his chopstick, I am thankful to my campers and students, their families, and my friends for helping me to affirm that this is the path I wish my life to follow.

Student Comments

I found that having a somewhat nonstandard essay helped a great deal in interviews. In almost all of my interviews I was able to discuss the experiences described in my essay in some depth. This way, I was walking on familiar ground and was not floored by a lot of tricky questions. That is, an interesting personal statement can promote a good discussion during interview.

Strengths

The essay has a great introduction. It is a feel-good story that makes the applicant immediately likable. The essay is very personal. The reasons the applicant is motivated to be a doctor are evidenced through his interactions with others.

Weaknesses

The essay doesn't include any experiences other than the role of counselor. While it is an endearing experience, it is discussed at great length and could have been shortened to make room for other experiences that may have prepared the applicant more directly for medical school. The essay is too long and probably would have benefited from an outline. The concluding paragraph should not have begun with "Thus."

ESSAY 9: Aerospace Engineering Ph.D. Candidate; Clinic Library Volunteer; Hospital ER Volunteer; Orthopedic Surgery Patient; Biomedical Research Experience; Leadership Skills and Awards
Accepted at: Harvard Medical School

Medicine and technology are becoming increasingly intertwined. The field has moved from the days of simple x-rays to implantable medication dispensers and gene therapy. Many illnesses thought incurable are now treatable due to a better understanding of the greatest machine ever engineered, the human body. However, medicine has a dual nature. Not only do physicians have to remedy the illness, but they must also treat the patient as a whole with regards to his pain and emotional well-being. As a result, the practice of medicine will forever be complex. I want to be a part of this challenging field, where discoveries are waiting to be made, so much research is needed, and application of research results can create visible and immediate changes.

To prepare for medical school, my college career has focused primarily on the engineering sciences. My educational background begins with undergraduate degrees, with honors, in aerospace and electrical engineering at the University of Minnesota. By attending classes year-round, I completed the degrees as well as my pre-medical course requirements within four years. Currently, I am pursuing a masters degree in aerospace engineering, with a focus on biomedical engineering, at the Massachusetts Institute of Technology. Continued study in this area leading to a Ph.D. is anticipated. While not firmly decided, my probable course of education will be to complete the first two years of medical school, finish my Ph.D. at MIT, and finally complete medical school. This track is standard for students pursuing M.D.'s and Ph.D.'s simultaneously. The medical specialty I intend to pursue has not been resolved. Given my educational history, aerospace medicine is a primary consideration. However, through recent personal experiences, I have become extremely interested in orthopedic surgery. I will likely maintain research interests in space medicine regardless of my eventual specialty.

I have had extensive exposure to "real" medicine, as a volunteer, medical professional, and patient. I began volunteering at the University of Minnesota Hospital and Clinic in 1994. My duties included delivering reading material to patients in the main surgery wards, the cancer wards, and the psychiatry clinics. Towards the end of my tenure at the U of MN, I was essentially in charge of the patient library. During the fall of 1995, I trained to become an emergency medical technician. Not only did the course provide me with additional health care skills, but I also gained an understanding of the roles of health care professionals other than physicians. Currently, I am a floor volunteer in the Massachusetts General Hospital Emergency Department (E.D.). My duties include: being the first hospital contact for walk-in patients, attending to immediate needs (such as bleeding, faintness, etc.) of walk-in patients, alerting the triage nurse to walk-in patients with life-threatening conditions, being a liaison between the E.D. staff and patient visitors, transporting patients to areas of the E.D. or hospital, attending to general patient comfort, delivering medical specimens to hospital laboratories, and assisting E.D. staff in any way they require. From these volunteer experiences, I have observed the importance and benefits of doctor-patient relationships and was given the opportunity to interact with many patients myself. I take comfort in the fact that I am helping to make a patient's stay at the hospital less traumatic. Often, I find myself listening to patients' concerns and helping to alleviate their fears. These interactions are more rewarding than I ever imagined. My own experiences as a hospital patient have had unexpected educational benefits. I have had two orthopedic surgeries and will have at least one more. From this exposure I have gained an understanding of what it is like to be a hospital patient, what it is like to be an orthopedic surgeon, how state-of-the-art diagnostic techniques are used, and some of the limitations of modern medicine. My volunteer and patient experiences have confirmed my decision to attend medical school.

Undoubtedly, my medical career will involve research. Already, I have participated in several biomedical research projects. To graduate with honors in both aerospace and electrical engineering, I completed two senior thesis projects. For my aerospace engineering major, I modeled nonuniformity of gas mixing in the lungs. My electrical engineering project was a preliminary design of an endoscope utilizing recent advancements in microelectronics for fluid dispensing. I am currently a research associate of MIT's Man-Vehicle Laboratory, a facility devoted to human performance in space. Few other schools or programs can offer comparable training for study in this interdisciplinary combination of aerospace engineering and the health sciences. My master's degree research topic is artificial gravity as a countermeasure to physiological space deconditioning. My emphasis is on the cardiovascular effects of using a short-arm centrifuge, which would create a gravity gradient along the body. Most likely, my Ph.D. topic will focus on treatments for disuse osteoporosis, a complication that affects astronauts, paralysis patients, and persons confined to bed rest. My course work at MIT has had a biomedical focus. As part of a medical devices course I completed in the spring of 1996, my partners and I designed an award-winning orthopedic device that improves diagnostic techniques for fracture fixation. My contribution was primarily assessing and promoting biocompatibility of the individual components and the device as a whole. Our design is patentable and we are continuing research during our extracurricular time.

Quality physicians are leaders in the health sciences and society. Through numerous academic and service oriented extracurricular activities, I have developed my leadership abilities. For a year I served as elected president of the University of Minnesota Institute of Technology (IT) Honors Group, an organization composed of the most academically talented students in IT. As a member of the IT Curriculum Committee, I participated in enhancing ITUs liberal education requirements so that students received a more well-rounded education. I was also a student representative to the IT Instructional Computing Committee, which was charged with deciding how to spend over one million dollars a year on computing equipment and services. As the elected Relations Director for the IT Student Board, the student government of IT, I had the responsibility of bringing student concerns to the attention of the administration and faculty. At MIT, I have resurrected graduate student concerns regarding a lack of a dental insurance plan, both through participation in the Graduate Student Council and as the graduate representative to the MIT Medical Advisory Committee. In addition, I have been aiding my advisor, Professor Laurence Young, with the MIT/Harvard bid for the National Space Biomedical Research Institute.

Regardless of where I attend medical school, I feel my future will entail medical practice and research that benefits patients as individuals and the field as a whole. My devotion to advancing medicine is sincere and I welcome the opportunity to prove myself.

Strengths

The essay contains a thorough description of the applicant's research projects and achievements.

Weaknesses

The essay is too long. The third and fourth paragraphs have obvious transitional areas where the applicant should have broken them into separate paragraphs. It is a dry and impersonal essay that contains a lot of information that should be (and is most likely) contained elsewhere in the application. He does not convincingly articulate why he wishes to become a doctor. He is obviously a bright and qualified candidate but he did not use the essay as an opportunity to reveal anything personal or particularly interesting about himself, so while this essay did not hurt him, it was not likely an asset to his application.

ESSAY 10: Motivation since Childhood; Unpleasant Doctor Experience; Goal to Be a Pediatrician; Swimming and Skiing Instructor; Volunteer Ski Patrol; Attempt to Save a Life with CPR; Musician and Singer

Accepted at: University of California—San Francisco School of Medicine; Johns Hopkins University School of Medicine; University of Washington School of Medicine; University of Rochester School of Medicine; Tufts University School of Medicine; Washington University School of Medicine; St. Louis University Health Sciences Center; Harvard Medical School

One day you will read in the National Geographic of a faraway land with no smelly bad traffic. In those green-pastured mountains of Fotta-fa-Zee everybody feels fine at a hundred and three 'cause the air that they breathe is potassium-free and because they chew nuts from the Tutt-a-Tutt Tree. This gives strength to their teeth, it gives length to their hair, and they live without doctors, with nary a care.
—Dr. Seuss, You're Only Old Once

Unfortunately for those of us inhabiting the non-Seussian world, this scenario is about as likely as encountering elephants perched on bird eggs or small furry orators standing atop tree stumps. The book goes on to describe treatment of a type that is seen all too often in our world of doctors. The hapless patient's experience in the clinic is, unfortunately, one that I have shared; it is in fact a driving force behind my motivation to become a physician. My experiences as a child have been instrumental in my current direction: I would like to become the pediatrician I never had. On numerous occasions I was ignored by my family physician simply because I was a child. I was obviously unaware of my body, or at least unable to express myself, since I was under five feet tall. When I walked into the office with my mother, he asked her how I felt, without ever sparing a glance for me (to which my mother generally replied, "Why don't you ask her?"). On those rare occasions on which he did deign to speak to me, it was to remind me of the sunny Saturday on which I was born and the picnic he had to leave because of my imminent arrival. As I grew older and began visiting the office without my parents,

103

he seemed at a loss—what to say to this person who was not yet of a respectable age? He soon settled on, "How are your parents? I still remember that Saturday. . . ." This was, and continues to be, extremely frustrating. Because of my love of and interest in a future career with children, I have sought work with them in several capacities. I have taught them, both as a swimming and skiing instructor. I have guided, watched, and played with them as a summer employee at a day care facility. I have learned much in the process about communicating with them. Time and again, my experience has shown me that, while they are in no way miniature adults, children most certainly are thinking human beings and deserve to be treated as such, although always on a level appropriate to their age.

Outside of my frustrations in the doctor's office, I have found other factors pointing me toward a career in medicine. As I pursued interests in athletics I found ways, sometimes rather unexpectedly, that medicine could take a part. I moved on from teaching skiing to become a volunteer member of the National Ski Patrol. In this way I was able to administer emergency medicine in a setting available to me as an avid skier and a student. I also worked for several summers as a lifeguard. I never really considered, however, that my training would prove so beneficial in my other leisure activities. One afternoon I was out horseback riding with my sister, who is also trained in first aid, when a person came running up the bridle trail. An elderly Parkinson's patient had fallen off a dam, and was gravely injured and in need of immediate aid. I had always assumed that my first real experience with CPR would be more sterile, using a mask and rubber gloves, not riding gloves, to protect me from blood-borne viruses. But this was as messy as it was real, and none of my training had quite prepared me for what I would experience: The exhilaration and single-minded determination to restore life to this person upon whom I had never before laid eyes. Unfortunately the afternoon did not end as we might have hoped; we were unable to resuscitate him. But the energy and spirit of teamwork surrounding those of us laboring to reclaim this man's life as we waited and waited for an ambulance to arrive were so strong as to be tangible, and called me as nothing ever had before. A heretofore nebulous inclination had become a decision: I wanted to get into this business of shaping lives, but on an extended basis during which I could get to know my patients and help them to maintain and restore their health over time, instead of only intervening when a crisis such as this occurred.

So I have spent my time, playing and singing, traveling and studying those topics that I'm interested in and that will help to shape the person who I am in the process of becoming. There hasn't been nearly enough time for everything I would love to do, but I have found, or more accurately made, time for as much as possible, with the knowledge that there is always more to learn, more to experience. Outside of academics, my major commitment is music, and through my playing and singing, I have been able to visit parts of the country and of the world that I would not otherwise have seen. I have been able to touch the lives of others and bring them joy as I myself have found joy in the dedication to a pursuit and the practice of a skill, not done by rote, but truly performed. This same dedication and love of learning will be invaluable to me as a physician, as will the many experiences which will help me to be more than merely a competent automaton or one of Seuss's "Oglers" who "silently, grimly [ogles] away" at patients, but a vibrant and caring physician. As I can hardly foresee a National Geographic description of a place in which we can live without doctors, I can only strive to be one of those doctors with whom we not only can but want to live.

Student Comments

I actually sat down one afternoon to write the essay; I hate lingering over things for too long. I have something of a history of quoting Dr. Seuss in essays, and my sister bet me that I wouldn't do it this time . . . so I did. I figured anywhere too uptight to not appreciate a very relevant reference was not somewhere I was interested in going.

Strengths

This is a personal essay that reveals a likeable personality to the admissions committee. The applicant tells interesting stories from her past and weaves them into an essay that adequately describes why she wants to become a doctor. She leaves academic achievements and research projects to other areas of her application.

Weaknesses

While overall this is a good essay, the applicant could have benefited from an edit. The content was solid but the writing skills could have been improved.

ESSAY 11: Medical Project Volunteer in Africa; Renal Research Lab Volunteer; Hospital Volunteer; Literature and Policy Background; Jazz Musician

Accepted at: University of California—San Francisco School of Medicine; Columbia University College of Physicians and Surgeons; Cornell University Medical College; Yale University School of Medicine; Stanford University School of Medicine; University of Pennsylvania School of Medicine; Duke University School of Medicine; Mount Sinai School of Medicine, CUNY; Harvard Medical School

As the rusted-out Land Rover made its way cautiously through dense thicket and crevices in the rocky dirt road, those of us sitting on top were able to peer through the trees at a sublime West African landscape. Our destination was S., a tiny village 300 miles upcountry where running water and electricity were unheard of. . . let alone access to basic health care. This was the summer of my freshman year at Brown, when I joined a multinational team on a medical development project in Sierra Leone. One afternoon a woman who had trekked many miles through the jungle to find care approached our clinic with an infant in her arms. She was not lactating effectively, and her child lay emaciated and dying. As I held the baby and administered a simple oral rehydration therapy and taught the mother to do the same, I was overcome with the sense of my relationship to this child and mother and by my ability to make a tangible difference in people's lives through the act of healing—the essence of being a physician.

My desire to become a doctor has developed through several years of academic, professional, and volunteer work as well as personal introspection. These have strengthened my conviction that through medicine I will be able to make a meaningful contribution to people's lives on both the individual and societal levels. Moreover, I hope that my various experiences will help me to be a broader, more informed, and more sensitive physician.

Reflecting on my endeavors, I see a common theme of humanitarian concern—a sensibility that grew out of early experiences living abroad with my family. As I became acquainted with myriad cultures, I developed an appreciation for the similarities and differences between societies. But more profoundly, witnessing vast basic needs in developing countries shaped my resolve to make a difference by serving others. Early on I looked to medicine as a means of doing so, and during high school I volunteered in a renal research lab. Joining daily rounds and visiting patients who would benefit from the research gave meaning to the work. I was also inspired by the positive impact that my father, a physician, had on people's lives.

At Brown and Oxford my interests in culture and in the difficulties of cross-cultural communication drew me to study the relationships between literature, society and politics. I discovered literature's unique ability to articulate the human connections that underlie cultural differences this provided an intellectual underpinning for my commitment to public service, particularly for my involvement in campus race relations issues. In addition, my studies of the sociopolitical components of underdevelopment taught me that improved infrastructure and health education might have prevented many of the conditions we had treated in Africa. I acted on my growing policy concerns by working with the U.S. State Department in Nigeria and at the B. Institution, where I gained firsthand insight into policy formulation.

But I soon realized that helping people in a direct and tangible way held greater meaning for me than did the arena of policy. When thinking seriously about a career path, my early interests in medicine were renewed as I reflected on how fulfilling my volunteer experiences had been, particularly working with patients in Sierra Leone and in a hospital context. I had also been inspired in Nigeria, seeing the contribution dedicated physicians made to the quality of people's lives in poor areas—and the acute need for doctors in underserved regions. And I recognized that within the field of health care policy, the input of experienced physicians is vital when designing programs. Acting on this decision, I served as an emergency room volunteer in Washington and applied to the Bryn Mawr Post Baccalaureate Program. At Bryn Mawr I have been struck by my flourishing interest in the scientific side of medicine, particularly molecular genetics, oncology and neurology. I have followed my clinical interests by volunteering at Hahnemann. This spring I will be returning to Sierra Leone with a grass-roots medical development organization to work setting up rural health clinics and to write a report outlining regional health care priorities.

A separate part of my life, my love for and involvement with music, has enhanced my appreciation for creativity and for the discipline of fine tuning a skill. An especially rewarding quality of music is the way it can forge connections between people: While touring Spain with a jazz ensemble we encountered a group of children with Down's Syndrome. At first they seemed detached, but when we played for them they became animated—dancing, laughing and smiling. Such experiences have impressed on me that relating to people is a vital component of healing.

This past year at Bryn Mawr has confirmed for me that medicine is a dynamic field in which I can bring together my interests in development policy and in serving people directly as a physician. I believe that the skills I have acquired through research, the study of literature, policy analysis, volunteer work, music and cross-cultural interaction will continue to develop within medicine and will enable me to make a meaningful contribution.

Strengths

The applicant describes interesting experiences in the essay that help reveal likeable aspects of her personality. Her humanitarian work is admirable and provides proof of her dedication and motivation to become a physician. She doesn't reflect on hard skills that can be found elsewhere in her application. Instead, she lets her soft skills shine, thus allowing the admissions committee to get to know her as a real person.

Weaknesses

The essay was not particularly well written from a grammatical perspective and included some obvious typos. It would have benefited from a stronger conclusion that did more than summarize points included in the essay.

Essay 12: Motivated since Childhood; Father's Influence; Health Care Debate; Tutor; Cardiac/Coronary Volunteer; Well-rounded Academic Background; Asian Studies; Authored High School Research Study Guide
Accepted at: Harvard Medical School

Since my childhood, my father's inspirational recounts as a cardiologist have captured my heart and my interest. While some have tried to sway me from becoming a doctor by noting the grim specter of health care reform looming overhead, I have found myself eager to participate in the public health care debate for the very same reasons I am drawn to enter the medical profession itself. In addressing society's urgent need for a more efficient and equitable health care system, health care reform centers around working to care and working to cure. To me, these two fundamental tenets infuse the medical profession like no other profession and serve as my principal motivations for pursuing this path. Through my experiences in academic exploration and community service, I have learned that I enjoy both the caring, personal interaction and the intellectual discovery in being a physician.

During my high school and college years, I have explored different areas of community service. Volunteering in the hospital setting and tutoring have been fulfilling experiences because, in both, I have had the opportunity to develop close, personal relationships with individuals in need and to help them during a critical stage of their life. In my freshman year I tutored geometry to an enthusiastic student at C. High School, and I am proud to say that I helped make a difference, not only in the final outcome of the course, but in his self-confidence and his attitude towards the field of mathematics. In my sophomore year I tutored for the English as a Second Language program in Boston's Chinatown. As a second generation Filipino-American, reaching out to the Chinatown community was a particularly rewarding experience for me because I knew my efforts would help open new opportunities for people who, like my parents and grandparents, immigrated to the United States.

I have also participated in the caring element of the medical profession, providing companionship to patients in the hospital setting. Throughout high school, I volunteered in the Coronary Care Unit and the Cardiac Rehabilitation Center at Mercer Medical Center, a hospital located in downtown Trenton, New Jersey. In the Coronary Care Unit, when patients needed help, I would assist them in tasks such as eating and moving about the hospital. In the Cardiac Rehabilitation Center, I helped nurses take and record the blood pressure and heart rate of patients. Much of the time, however, was spent conversing with the patients and getting to know them better. I realized through my close contact with patients, physicians, and nurses that I would enjoy working in the health care setting, reaching out to those who were sick, and making the lifetime commitment to "be there" for those in need. I continued to volunteer in the hospital setting when I came to Harvard, this time addressing the important, but sometimes forgotten, needs of the families visiting patients. Spending my Saturday afternoons working in the family waiting area of the Coronary Care Unit at Massachusetts General Hospital, I served as a non-medical liaison to expedite communication between the busy CCU staff and the visitors, provided non-medical information to the families on the nature and location of hospital services, and offered peer support to the often anxious family members. Volunteering in the CCU waiting area helped me realize that the suffering caused by sickness afflicts, not only the patients, but their family members as well, and provided me a unique opportunity to gain experience in caring for their needs.

It would be simplistic for me to say that I have chosen to devote my life to the medical profession only because I have a strong desire to help people. All jobs, in their own way, contribute to society, and quite a few involve the establishment of personal relationships, including teaching. But to me, only one profession also has the dynamism of continuous intellectual exploration—medicine. In an era in which rapid technological progress and health care reform continuously transform the study, practice, and ethics of medicine, working to cure requires a passion for learning and discovery, and I have found that I thrive on this intellectual exploration. For me, it is a wonderful feeling to make an intellectual leap and manage to land feet first upon a convincing conclusion, or to be able to weave once disparate pieces of information into a coherent synthesis, and, after stepping back to observe the big picture, to be able to trace the pivotal themes running throughout. The moment of realization that, through time and effort, an enigma has been solved and my vision has been deepened and expanded, is a great thrill which never fails to leave me thirsting for the next challenge.

The excitement of intellectual discovery has encouraged me to explore a number of fields. While my major is biochemistry, my academic interests also encompass Asian studies, languages, music, computer science, health care, and environmental policy; as a result, prioritizing my academic goals while at Harvard has proven a challenge in itself. Because of the ongoing trade disputes between the United States and Japan, the recent dynamism of the Four Little Dragons (Singapore, Hong Kong, Taiwan, and Korea), and my Asian heritage, when I came to Harvard I decided to delve deeper into the field of Asian culture. I have taken advantage of the strong Asian studies department at Harvard, studying Japanese and the industrialization of East Asia, researching the role of the Japanese primary school system in socialization, and examining the role of the Japanese government in promoting economic growth. In the field of health care, I have researched family planning programs in the developing world and the relationship between health care and human rights in the context of the AIDS epidemic. In addition, I have managed to fit courses in chamber music and computer programming into my schedule, but my passion for classical music and interests in environmental policy have remained largely unfulfilled. The demands of the clock have forced me to relegate my studies in these areas to activities outside of class, such as playing Debussy on the pianos in Paine Hall or researching sustainable development as Director of the Model United Nations Development Programme.

My rewarding experiences in growing intellectually have not only fueled my own passion for exploration and discovery, but have inspired me to share my enthusiasm for learning with others, particularly in the field of science. Working together with the faculty at my high school, I have helped reform the science curriculum in an attempt to shift the focus from the accumulation of background material to exploration—from details and data to dynamism and discovery—by restoring the critical balance between theory and experiment. To help high school students embark on their own exciting voyages to understand the world around us, I wrote a study guide describing how to approach scientific research and titled it Frontier to emphasize exploration and intellectual discovery. Students at The Lawrenceville School currently use Frontier in the new program, and Research Corporation of Tucson, Arizona has recently published the study guide.

To me, there is only one profession which satisfies both my curiosity and my desire to help those in need. Incorporating both the caring, personal, physician-patient relationship and the dynamism of continuous learning, the medical profession is the profession I eagerly embrace, and I believe it is also the best way I can harness my own talents and abilities for the benefit of others.

Strengths

The applicant relates many applicable volunteer experiences in a well-structured and well-written essay.

Weaknesses

This is a standard personal statement to medical school. It has all the necessary ingredients but it was not particularly interesting or memorable. Though many volunteer experiences were shared, they were not actually discussed on a personal level. The inclusion of extracurricular activities and academic pursuits could have made a bigger impact if they had been woven into a story from the applicant's past, thereby allowing the admissions committee to get to know him a little better.

ESSAY 13: Childhood/Family Experiences; Religious Church of Jesus Christ of Latter-day Saints; Unpleasant Medical Experience; Interest in Alternative Approaches; Well-rounded Academic Background; Exercise-Science Major; Financially Self-supported

Accepted at: Harvard Medical School

"One time, a family cat captured. . . a moth. The cat's play disturbed E., who promptly got a local veterinarian on the phone to get tips on reviving the mortally wounded moth. The moth didn't make it, but knowing E.'s enthusiasm, Mrs. E. is more optimistic about the park." (*The Idaho Statesman*, 11/22/78)

This article, about me as a ten-year-old boy trying to turn a nearby drainage pond into a park, had a misprint—it was a mouse, not a moth. Still, this example shows why people have always said I would probably be a doctor or veterinarian. Wandering the fields, I brought home sick and hurt creatures; if anyone found an injured bird or animal, they brought it to me for care.

We didn't exactly live on a farm, but were in farming country. My father always made sure that we had a large garden; that, along with a small vineyard, orchard and corn field, provided work for us six kids and a little extra family income. My parent's couldn't give us allowances and we had to help pay for our own clothes, so we worked on local farms (bucking hay bales, moving sprinkler pipes, etc.) and did whatever we could find—I started an early morning daily paper route (on my bike, in all weather) at age eleven, and had it for five years.

During this period, we did manage to find time for other things. Besides earning the rank of Eagle Scout, I sang in school choirs, performed in state piano boards, acted in school and community theater, ran (and earned a letter) in cross-country and track (until forced by my Junior year to choose between school sports and earning money), and served as a student body representative in my high school.

After two semesters at Boise State, I volunteered to serve for two years as a missionary with the Church of Jesus Christ of Latter-day Saints, going to the California, Ventura Mission. I loved it, learned a lot, being able to dedicate every hour to helping and teaching people of all nationalities, cultures and religions. Many of the friends I made among the people and the other missionaries are still very close, and the lessons I learned from all of my experiences affect my life every day.

Returning to school, my classes included math and sciences (subjects I had shied away from before)—out of curiosity, at first; then, to keep my options open. I actually enjoyed them, and managed to get good grades. My love for the humanities continued, including writing guest editorials and articles for the Fullerton College school paper, and I was awarded the annual Book Award for Excellence in Foreign Language from the Spanish department. My activities were rounded out by helping at a nearby adolescent rehabilitation clinic, and serving the single members of my church as the activities committee chairman and representative to the regional council.

In high school, I had had some health problems and seen a number of doctors. When a general practitioner didn't find anything, he sent me to a specialist, who sent me to another, who sent me to another. . . none of whom could find a problem, yet all of whom charged my parents what seemed exorbitant fees.

This experience soured me on the medical profession. My interests in people continued to grow, but because of my cynicism toward physicians and lack of money, medical school wasn't seriously considered. Besides, math and sciences didn't appeal to me at that time like music, drama, philosophy and writing did.

I pursued psychology and the humanities, while growing more fascinated by health, nutrition, and what people I knew had found in "alternative" approaches to health, including preventive and Eastern medicine. Although a natural skeptic, it seemed to me that if something appears to work for rational, respectable people, it should be taken seriously—researched, to determine whether the benefit is merely psychological or not—contrary to the doctors I had met, who felt that if THEY didn't have it, it was "dangerous". This seemed narrow-minded, opposing the principles I understood "science" to be based upon.

Upon transferring to USC, I found that my view of the medical establishment wasn't really accurate—there ARE those who care more about helping people than about the money or their intellectual pride. As a result, I've decided to enter medical school, focusing on research and preventive medicine. My major in Exercise Science is providing a strong background in physiology and nutrition.

Throughout my college career, I have had to support myself financially. Working full-time while at Boise State as a restaurant manager, and then doing singing telegrams, fitness consulting, and running my own window-cleaning business since moving to California have allowed me to get by. Now, my work-study research job at the LA County General Hospital/USC Health Sciences Campus is also providing excellent experience in working in both hospital and research settings. My church responsibilities continually mean opportunities for volunteer service, and as Vice-President of the USC chapter of S. fraternity, one of my projects has been setting up and directing our relationship with Challengers, a local inner-city youth club with which our fraternity is now involved in activities and tutoring.

Strengths

The essay has an entertaining story in the beginning that immediately pulls the reader in. This is a humble and likeable applicant who has a lot to offer. We know this not because he spells it out for us, but because we can draw conclusions from his diverse experiences. His stories from childhood are evidence of his focus and his hard-working nature, qualities that will serve him well in medical school.

Weaknesses

The essay would have benefited from an edit because it contains typos and lacks a conclusion. Both issues would have been corrected if the applicant had sought feedback—resulting in a much stronger essay.

ESSAY 14: Electric Engineering Background; Biomedical Engineering Research; Radiology Research Assistant; ER and Geriatrics Hospital Volunteer; Student Advisor; Editor and Scriptwriter
Accepted at: Harvard Medical School

To heal and to comfort, these are the goals I share with physicians, past and present. Tomorrow's physicians, I believe, will have an even better opportunity to attain the goal of healing through technological breakthroughs, of which magnetic resonance imaging and gene therapy are examples we have seen in recent years. However, I also believe that physicians must always be the compassionate bringers of hope, as no amount of technology will ever replace physicians' sensitivity to their patients' needs. Ever since I was a child, I have had a strong interest in science and technology. At the same time, my enthusiasm for working with people and desire to help others have guided my activities in college and beyond. Together, these qualities have shaped my decision to study medicine.

As an undergraduate at Cornell University, I majored in electrical engineering. Initially, I was drawn to this field because its rigorous and broad curriculum would give me a solid foundation in the physical sciences. However, as I explored beyond the elegance of its underlying theories, I was fascinated by how the application of electronics has affected people's lives. Therefore, I decided to spend some time in the industry. Under the auspices of the Engineering Cooperative Program at Cornell, I worked for B in North Carolina for eight months during my junior year. This experience proved to be very rewarding. As a software engineering intern, I saw how the combination of my personal skills and technical knowledge enabled both workers outside my department and customers of the company to understand the practical implications of our work. In turn, they taught me the relevance of theirs. Among the most important lessons I learned was that advancement in technology must be built upon social considerations—technology developed in isolation from human concerns and without regard to its limitations is doomed for rejection.

Upon my return to Cornell for my senior year, I decided to pursue research work with more direct human applications. Under the guidance of Professor B., I successfully used artificial neural networks to distinguish normal electrocardiogram patterns from abnormal ones, including those that result from pre-ventricular contractions and ST segment depressions. Following an independent investigation, I also explained the phenomenon known as 'bursting', whereby artificial neural networks avalanche into a region of very large errors. Armed with this experience in biomedical engineering research, I decided to spend a year after graduating from Cornell in the department of radiology at the J. As a research assistant for Professor M. and Dr. Z., I am using spin tagged magnetic resonance images and computer tomographical techniques to reconstruct the three-dimensional motion of the myocardium. We are confident that the information that yields from these studies will allow cardiologist to diagnose more quickly and accurately the extent and severity of ischemia in patients.

While my interest in biomedical technology stems from my academic background, my determination to pursue a career in medicine has been driven by my clinical experience as a volunteer in the emergency departments of the D. and the J., and in the geriatrics department at the T. in Ithaca. During the dramatic episodes I witnessed in the emergency room, I realized that the analytical skills which I have developed as an engineer will be central to the diagnosis and treatment of patients. What I cherished most of all while working in these hospitals, however, was the unique opportunity to comfort patients. Through the odd smile from the patient who was in pain and the passing "thank you" from the disoriented patient, I caught a glimpse of the tremendous emotional satisfaction which the power to comfort holds. Although some of the patients I came into contact with were somewhat abusive and confrontational, I did my best to help, knowing that their physical ailment and fear, and not the patients themselves, were the source of their ill-temper. My time spent volunteering at hospitals was as educational as it was emotionally rewarding—in working with elderly patients, I came to learn that companionship and patience can often be the best healing tools.

Beyond my clinical activities, I have tried to strengthen my communication and personal skills, skills which are essential to the practice of any medical speciality. As an engineering ambassador, I have interacted regularly with prospective engineering students and their parents at Cornell. In leading tours and discussion panels, I have striven to be tactful and, at the same time, truthful in answering their questions about Cornell. During my time as an engineering student advisor, I counseled distressed freshmen who were having difficulties coping with the academic pressures at Cornell. Such experience taught me how one's psychological pain can be relieved by another's concern and care. I also experimented with teaching, and tutored English grammar to an adult high-school student when I was in North Carolina. The experience turned out to be both challenging and fun, as I learned that the art of teaching lies in flexibility and persuasion. On the literary front, I have been actively involved in the editorial work of the Compass Magazine at Cornell, a forum devoted to international issues. I also co-authored the scripts used in a cultural show sponsored by Cornell's HKSA for two years. Although my background in script writing and stage design was initially limited, I took full advantage of this learning experience, which I thoroughly enjoyed, especially when my humor on paper was translated into laughter in the audience.

The practice of medicine, I believe, will also be a learning experience for me, as I continually draw upon my background in technology and commitment towards people, to find more effective ways to treat my patients. Following my graduation from medical school, I hope to pursue this work through research fellowships in a hospital setting, where I shall be best able to combine research with patient care. While the advancement of medical technology might entail many challenges, I am confident that, with perseverance, I will succeed in my undertaking to heal and to comfort.

Strengths

This is a well-written essay that adequately explains the applicant's motivation to become a doctor. He effectively describes how his education and research in the hard sciences have come together with his volunteer experiences in the medical field to lead him down a path toward medical school. Through his discussions, he comes across as intelligent and qualified.

Weaknesses

For all its merits, this essay is still lacking something. Most simply put, it is dry and not particularly fun to read. These factors make it unmemorable. The applicant describes a lot of extracurricular activities but his descriptions aren't personal accounts. Instead of revealing them through stories, he writes quick descriptions of many experiences and doesn't manage to unveil his character in an engaging and cohesive essay.

ESSAY 15: Motivated by an Accident; ER Volunteer; Camp Counselor and Big Brother; Health Center Medical Assistant
Accepted at: Harvard Medical School

Ironically, the first time I seriously considered becoming a doctor was as a patient. One night in August in 1989, trying to catch-up to my campers, I ran, slipped, and crashed through a glass door. I was rushed to a hospital to repair the four tendons I had severed. Initially, I did not know what would happen to me or to the use of my hand. After the surgical resident examined me and told me that I would be fine with surgery and rehabilitation, I felt relieved. He had not yet laid a hand on me, but his words did wonders for my spirits. During my recovery, I imagined how good it would be to help others the way this young physician had helped me. It would feel good, I thought, to have my patients return to thank me for the care I had provided. Undoubtedly, this anticipated glory was a large part of my attraction to medicine.

I became an Emergency Room volunteer at the Wellesley Hospital in downtown Toronto so as to gain some first-hand experience as a care provider. I realized quickly that my vision of life in medicine was distorted. In my fantasy, patients never died and doctors never dealt with failure. Patients were relatively healthy and well motivated. In reality, many of the patients were elderly and could not take care of themselves. Others were addicted to drugs and did not seem to care about their health. The ER was overcrowded and the staff overworked. Some patients cursed or spat at the staff while others left without waiting to be seen. In any case, there were few "thank yous," no grateful smiles and no glory. I wondered whether it was all worth the sacrifice.

Among the newly discovered drawbacks, however, there were unexpected rewards. I remember vividly one man who came into the Wellesley Hospital emergency room during the winter of 1994. Brought in by the police after attempting suicide, he sat in the interview room sobbing with his head resting in his blood-stained hands. When I fearfully sat next to him, he told me about the contempt his family had for him. Realizing that I could do little for him, I sat and listened while he talked. After a few minutes, my fear gave way to interest. We first talked about his family and then about literature and film. I learned a lot that day by listening and trying to learn about his life. That was the first time I had taken time to listen; not just to what he wanted to eat or drink, but about his fears, his pain, and his joy. I cannot ascertain how helpful I was. I did not tend to his wounds, nor did I repair his relationship with his family. But I did help him feel human for an hour or two. There was something warm about forming a bond, albeit a temporary one.

The opportunity to learn from others' stories—their successes and their failures—is a privilege many take for granted. Luckily, through my positions as camp counsellor and program director, medical assistant, and "big brother," I have had numerous opportunities to listen and learn. By embarking on a career in medicine, I hope to continue that learning. As Dr. R. writes, "we chose this life because it lets us know people. . .we chose to become doctors because we would have patients*."

Although many professions allow for some degree of personal interaction, medicine appeals to me in addition on an intellectual level. Through my work as a medical assistant at the Health Center at Cornell and my externship positions with a number of physicians, I learned of the opportunity for "detective" work. I relish the prospect of working with patients and collecting clues from such sources as personal histories, physical exams, and laboratory tests. By nurturing personal bonds and asking the proper questions, physicians have an opportunity to delve into the human soul and learn more about each individual. The advantage clinicians have over other professionals is their skill in collecting information from biological, psychological, and sociological perspectives and merging them to paint a more complete portrait of each patient.

It is these portraits that make life as a physician both colorful and daunting because they not only bring doctors closer to the people they treat, they bring them closer to their pateints' pain and uncertainty. No training and practice can make that experience easy. Weighing the costs and benefits, however, I believe it will be worth the sacrifice.

*Quotation taken from "To Listen, To Recognize" reprinted from The Pharos of Alpha Omega Alpha, Fall 1986, 49 (4), pp. 10-13.

Strengths

This is a good essay. It is brief, personal, and interesting. The applicant takes a decisive step away from her application and uses the essay as an opportunity to sell herself to the admissions committee. She knows that her achievements and coursework are well documented elsewhere so she doesn't replicate them in her essay. She utilizes her personal and volunteer experiences to tell stories that reveal the thoughtfulness that she has put into her decision to become a doctor.

Weaknesses

The essay doesn't have any real weaknesses. However, it could have been an even stronger asset to her application if the applicant had seamlessly included some measures of success into her stories.

ESSAY 16: High School Teacher with AIDS; SCID/Genetics Research Experience; HIV Counselor

Accepted at: University of California—San Diego School of Medicine; University of Pennsylvania School of Medicine; Jefferson Medical College, Thomas Jefferson University; Temple University School of Medicine; Harvard Medical School

Before I found out that my high school Spanish teacher was HIV-positive, AIDS was not much more than a bunch of statistics to me. The disease, its course, and the people afflicted with it seemed alien to my life—as distant as the continent from which the virus was supposed to have sprung. Then Mr. T. stopped coming to school. When he reappeared a few months later to wish us well on the advanced placement exam, his face looked sallow. His voice, once a thunderous bass that rumbled in class and reverberated down the hallway, was weak and thin. Seeing my teacher looking so unfamiliar was my shocking introduction to AIDS. I felt as if I were in the presence of a stranger, this mysterious disease, who was insulting Mr. T. right in front of my eyes. I wanted to know who this stranger was.

I entered college, believing that biology could explain to me why life's processes went awry. I learned that the body is exquisitely complex, but I was reassured by the underlying theme of systems. Even if I didn't know all the molecules and connections, there seemed no denying that a fundamental order existed.

From physiology to cell biology to molecular genetics, my classes presented smaller and smaller systems to explain the origins of diseases. Finally, in genes, with their innocuous four letter alphabet, I felt I was learning the foundation of it all. If biology provided the keys to understanding life, then genetics must be the master key (if only we could see some of the doors we were trying to open). During two summers in a research laboratory at The Children's Hospital of Philadelphia, I helped track down the gene causing X-linked severe combined immunodeficiency (SCID).

Even though AIDS and SCID are very different diseases (SCID is exclusively hereditary), each compromises the body's defense mechanisms against foreign pathogens. I felt this was a significant connection. In

SCID, I was meeting a distant cousin of AIDS. Learning about common themes of immunodeficiency disorders, such as the perils of opportunistic infections, helped me to begin to understand what had happened to Mr. T. In the SCID laboratory, and in classroom seminars on infectious diseases, science was helping me demystify disease.

In the same year that Mr. T. became ill, my grandfather died during bypass surgery and my father underwent chemotherapy and radiation treatment for colon cancer. Since then, disease has had a human face for me. To better understand how people deal with disease or the fear of disease, I've become a volunteer counselor in an HIV clinic.

Speaking to people who come in for free testing, I've found that discussing HIV, getting the scary words (and acronyms) out in the open, is a way for many people to release their anxiety. Through expression in their own words, they make the disease real, which helps them to see that it is also preventable. Then, they often take the next step, making specific goals to maintain their health, whether they are HIV-negative or positive. What science in class and lab did for me in confronting the difficult issues of AIDS, talk does for my clients.

As an HIV counselor in an anonymous clinic, I feel both the potential of my role and its limits. I can't go home with my clients to remind them to keep condoms under the bed, but I can help them make a plan—something that could stay with them much longer than the information I offer. At the end of one session, one client surprised me with his response to a question I had asked: "What do you think you'll do with the HIV information?" There was a silence in the counseling room as the client pondered, but I recall sensing the comfort of the silence. This was a session that seemed to be producing the potential for a breakthrough (not every session does), and I waited patiently. He responded, "I think I'll ask my girlfriend to use her own needles." Then, the client thanked me for having asked the question.

I was thrown. My client proposed a strategy for reducing his HIV risk, but he didn't address what was likely his main issue—heroin use. Should I validate his plan? In effect, that's what I did, because I didn't challenge the drug issue. When he left the clinic, I practically wanted to follow him out the door. I wondered if I would ever see him again and be able to ask him how his plan was going. I wondered if he would ultimately seek help for his drug use. My supervisor reminded me that I had done my job as an HIV counselor. I had helped the client make a plan; he had even thanked me for it.

And I can thank him in return. He reminded me that although I have worked to understand disease in the classroom, the laboratory, and the clinic, I still have much to learn about caring for all aspects of a patient's health. I am eager to continue the learning process in the New Pathway Program at Harvard Medical School.

Student Comments

I spent about three weeks writing my essay sending it back and forth to my sister, who is a writer/editor. I feel that my essay was very important to my application because my grades were not so stellar (I have C's on my transcript) but I had some life experience (from being out of school for three years) which was unique. I was very conscious to write the essay from a humble perspective, as I've read essays with many "I" sentences, and to me they sound very pompous.

Strengths

This is a great essay. The applicant begins the essay with an interesting (and heart-wrenching) story. She connects it to her pursuit of premedical studies, her research, and eventually to her work as an AIDS counselor. In doing so, she demonstrates her initial motivation and continued dedication toward a career in medicine. Through her work experience, she reveals her compassion for patients and a concern for their long-term health. She writes from a very personal perspective, allowing the admissions committee to get to know her. Her efforts paid off because, as the applicant notes, her application was not that stellar. Yet, through this personal essay, she stood out to the admissions committees and ultimately was accepted to many of the nation's best medical schools.

Weaknesses

None.

ESSAY 17: Sea Education Association Experience; Clinic and ER Volunteer; Health Care Intern; Math Background
Accepted at: University of Virginia School of Medicine; Harvard Medical School; University of Rochester School of Medicine

The Southern Cross hung low on the horizon at 3:00 a.m. as I came on deck for my watch. The 125' schooner Westward was hove-to, collecting deep-water samples over the mid-Atlantic ridge. Suddenly, a dramatic squall transformed the quiet deck into an organized frenzy of activity. My watchmates and I moved swiftly, closing up hatches, battening down and hauling the scientific equipment aboard. Within minutes the stars disappeared, the winds gusted to Force 7 and a black wall of rain trounced us. The elements were capricious, but during the blow, the choreography of teamwork was clear.

I was working as a deckhand with 20 students and 10 crew aboard a research vessel run by the Sea Education Association (SEA). The 2 1/2 month trans-Atlantic passage was a chance for the ship's company to work hard together, to lead and let others lead in turn, and to experience life in its fullest as we pitched in 15 foot swells or hauled up meter nets by moonlight. The community aboard Westward was close and teamwork imperative. There was no escaping the grueling task of setting the fisherman sail, the smelly chore of scrubbing the galley mats, or the short temper of a grumpy shipmate. Yet, I felt completely engaged. Like a physician working in a hospital, I rose to the demands of a rolling schedule, enduring mental and physical fatigue amid the stern necessity of the work at hand. Life at sea is full of unforgiving challenges and it was satisfying to exercise my mind, muscle and judgment to help sail the vessel safely on her way. I want to use the SEA experience as a template for the rest of my life and embark on a medical career that will be similarly intense and challenging.

Both at sea and on land, I have found great pleasure in the rewards of upholding and enriching the worlds of which I am a part. Editing my high school paper was a delicate project; it required tact, good judgment and consensus building as my co-editor and I resolved a brewing censorship dispute between our assistant editors and the school's administration. At Yale, a strong sense of community led me to a deep involvement in the activities of my residential college as a veteran member of the college council, director of intramural sports, and chairman of a record-breaking fundraising drive. Though I have not campaigned aggressively for leadership roles, my concern for constructive leadership and my reliable attitude have placed me in positions of responsibility.

My decision to become a physician has been percolating for several years. In a busy hallway in New York's Babies Hospital, I watched a young doctor hunker down to speak at eye level to a scared five-year-old and gently part a curtain of pain and fear in order to assess and treat a wound. Immediately I recognized the value and success of the doctor's approach, one I would like to apply as a healer. In Seattle, I volunteered in two contrasting medical settings: A low-income neighborhood clinic serving the elderly and the emergency room of a private pediatric hospital. Escorting an old man home from day-surgery and holding a toddler during a painful procedure helped focus my interest in medicine. Later, as I followed an internist and a pediatrician in adolescent medicine around their clinical practices in Boston, I was drawn to the myriad issues, some medical by many societal, that are subsumed in the physician-patient relationship. This summer, as an intern for Senator Kennedy's health care staff, I learned to respect the complexity of these policy issues.

I enjoy using my mind to solve tough problems. Majoring in math at Yale was an expression of this desire for intellectual challenge and rigor.

Now, I want to use this energy in a less abstruse and more practical context. Medicine merges my skills and interests; it is a chance to bring everything—analytical reasoning, sensory awareness, social conscience, teamwork, compassion—into the arena. I felt this fusion in the emergency room at Hahnemann University in Philadelphia. There an intern demonstrated the pleasure of working on medical problems, since they come attached to individuals who stand to benefit from the intellectual endeavor. I see the road ahead as a humbling one, however, for being with a patient struggling to heal is also a journey in self-discovery and in confronting one's own pain. I embrace the challenge.

Student Comments

I stewed over this essay for a while as I tried to succinctly incorporate many of the experiences that had led me to chose a career in medicine. It was important to me to tell a story, and to let the reader discover me through my descriptions of my experiences rather than by laying out personal qualities in a flat-footed way.

Strengths

This is an adequate personal statement that meets most of the expectations of an application essay. The applicant opens with an interesting story. Although the story has nothing to do with medicine or the applicant's pursuit of a career in it, he immediately grabs the attention of the reader by reliving an experience from his past that is obviously important to him.

Weaknesses

The applicant manages to pack a lot into this essay but he should have paid more attention to transitions and may have benefited from an outline, which would have allowed him to create a more cohesive essay. The third paragraph that discusses a few undergraduate and some high school activities does little to help the essay. The subjects are not discussed with much detail nor are they discussed from a perspective that is personal enough to make them interesting. It is not advisable to dip into high school for extracurricular activities unless you are able to weave them into a story that tells the admission committee a lot about who you are today.

ESSAY 18: Motivated by Childhood Illness; Career Switcher; Broadcasting Experience; HIV Research; Social Science and Communication Background

Accepted at: University of California—Los Angeles School of Medicine; Stanford University School of Medicine; University of Michigan Medical School; Washington University School of Medicine; Duke University School of Medicine; University of Pennsylvania School of Medicine; Harvard Medical School; University of Washington School of Medicine; Medical College of Wisconsin

My work experiences—ranging from public health projects in rural Latin America to work at urban battered women's shelters to peer counseling on a college campus—reflect my concern for people's "health" in a broad sense of the word. Yet I never imagined as an undergraduate in the social sciences that I would eventually become a doctor. I also never expected to call rehydration salts "anti-witch" treatment, but suddenly, one day, that made perfect sense.

The morning of New Year's day, 1978, was bright and sunny. Refreshed from a good night's sleep, I lifted the blankets, rose to my feet, and collapsed, unable to walk. Soon afterwards, emergency room doctors assured me that it was only a temporary viral infection and not, as my parents worried, a handicapping case of polio. I recovered from that frightening infection, but imprinted in my mind is the feeling of relief I felt at the hospital, where I could be confident about the professionals looking after me. This experience prompted me to consider dedicating my life to becoming a doctor, helping others, and giving them the same confidence I felt in that emergency room. Caring for my arthritis-afflicted mother for the past several years and volunteering at a local hospital have helped me realize that I have the compassion that motivates me to become a medical professional.

Despite having various interests, I have carefully determined to pursue an M.D.-Ph.D. program. My experiences have led me to believe that I will make an effective clinical physician since I enjoy working with people one-on-one, but that my other talents can be used to make even more far-reaching contributions to medicine and to society. As a newsroom teleprompter operator, I have been exposed to broadcasting and realize that I would enjoy delivering reports as a medical correspondent. I see the need for qualified medical personnel in the media to function as interpreters of medical knowledge for the general public. Though this is an option, my experiences in research have helped me decide to seek a career primarily as a scientific investigator.

My transcript and various awards, which include the UW Dean's Medal for the Sciences, demonstrate my academic ability, but research has been the most satisfying component of my undergraduate education. It has allowed me to develop my intellectual curiosity by applying learned

123

knowledge to new situations. For the last two years, I have been characterizing particular site-specific mutations in the envelope glycoprotein of the Human Immunodeficiency Virus (HIV) under the supervision of Dr. S. My planning and performing of experiments, collection of results, and conducting of extensive literature searches were brought together into a cohesive whole as my honors senior thesis, which was selected as the best undergraduate paper in Microbiology and awarded the J. Ordal Award. The results of my work are presented in a manuscript which is being submitted for publication. Also, I have contributed to a poster abstract at a recent international AIDS vaccines conference.

Since I would like to practice in both the clinic and the lab and therefore need to be much more than just a technician, I am currently completing a second degree in Speech Communication. Effective communication is crucial in all aspects of our lives, but particularly for physicians, who must be especially sensitive to the needs of their patients in the clinic and must be able to communicate clearly with colleagues as scientists. The opportunities I have had to develop interpersonal and public speaking skills are directly relevant to helping me become a better clinician and researcher.

Although completing two degrees and working have demanded much time, I have not allowed them to hinder my participation in activities which have helped me mature as a person. Serving as a counselor for junior-high youths in our church, leading bible studies, and operating the closed-circuit camera during Sunday services have given me important lessons about working with people. Studying piano for twelve years and learning tennis as a new sport have taught me the value of perseverance, dedication, and self-discipline. All of these activities, especially doubles tennis, have helped me become a better team player.

Wanting to become a doctor is not a recent desire, but a result of experiences over my lifetime. My willingness to work hard and to persevere through difficult and demanding situations, as well as my ability to relate to others will enhance my capacity to contribute to society as a doctor. Equally important, however, is that I expect to be satisfied as a research and clinical physician, intellectually challenged and content knowing that I am doing my best to help others.

Student Comments

This essay actually took me several weeks (on-and-off, of course) of writing. I felt that giving details about how my interest in medicine developed over time would set my essay apart from those of applicants who just simply stated that they wanted to "help others." I think the most difficult aspect of the writing process was trying to emphasize what I thought were my strong selling points without bragging, and I believe giving detailed examples helped in this regard.

Strengths

This essay contains a lot of information about the applicant including work experience, a personal story from childhood, research projects, hobbies, and interests. It was an adequate personal statement that did not hurt the applicant's chances of being accepted.

Weaknesses

Despite the fact that this applicant was accepted to medical school, this essay did not likely enhance his or her application. With the exception of the childhood illness, it reads like a prose CV. It would not be surprising if the applicant, instead of creating an outline, wrote down a lot of experiences and achievements that were to be noted in the essay and simply found a way to cram them all in. Unfortunately, the result was not a memorable essay.

ESSAY 19: Community Health Volunteer in Haiti; International Development and Public Health Background
Accepted at: Dartmouth Medical School; Brown University School of Medicine; Emory University School of Medicine; Harvard Medical School

"Dawn, do you believe in las brujas?" In witches?! I was just concluding a workshop on diarrhea and dehydration with a group of community health workers. In the border region between the Dominican Republic and Haiti it is commonly believed that the symptoms of dehydration are a result of children being "sucked by witches." So I diplomatically answered that although where I grew up people don't tend to believe in witches, undeniably there are places where individuals are more strongly influenced by the powers of magic. Apparently encouraged by my response, the women—who I trained and supervised as part of a mother-infant health program—proceeded to recount numerous tales of children's lives being saved by curanderos, or witch doctors, after having been "sucked."

In my mind, I was scrambling for a way to salvage our discussion of hygiene and oral rehydration. After listening carefully to their stories, I pointed out that despite the wide variety of rituals, prayers and herbs used to free the victim of witches, each of the "cures" they described involved the administration of liquids. They were soon deciding that whether a mother chooses to believe that her child has been affected by witches or by bacteria, it is always important to rehydrate the child. We concluded the meeting saying that when appropriate, properly prepared oral rehydration salts could be utilized as "anti-witch" treatment.

The complexity of human health has led me to the study of medicine. At the time of that training, my background included a degree in international development and experience working on community health programs in several countries. I expected that my next academic pursuit would be a masters in public health. However, along with increased exposure to the field, came the realization that I wanted more.

I wanted to be able to do more. While aware of the enormous value of health instruction and disease prevention, I found myself often feeling frustrated with the limitations of what I had to offer. People benefit from education and training, but at times they also need medicines and treatment. My efforts to help people improve their quality of life could be enhanced by expanding my capabilities. The study of medicine would greatly increase the impact that I could have on people's health.

I also wanted to know and understand more. Less altruistic than a desire to help others—yet an equally powerful motivating force in my life—is my love of learning. I have always found that for work to be truly satisfying to me, it must be intellectually stimulating. To conduct an effective health education campaign, one must learn to communicate information in a simplistic fashion, yet my own questions about health issues were increasingly complex. I wasn't content just knowing that diarrhea leads to dehydration; I was wondering how and why and what could be done to treat it and how does that work? With minimal preparation in the sciences, the challenge of entering a new academic field was enticing. Medical knowledge would afford me a much broader perspective on human health.

If both the physiology of dehydration and the belief that a child is being "sucked by witches" can be understood, then a person's health needs will be more effectively met. I now intend to study both medicine and public health, since I feel that an inter-disciplinary approach is best suited for confronting multifaceted health problems.

Student Comments

It took me a few months to write and revise the essay. I gave it to lots of people—both knowledgeable of the med school application process and not—to read and criticize. I think that my essay was a very significant part of my application, since in all of my interviews the story I related was a prominent topic of conversation. I know people have been hearing this since they applied to college, but the first sentence is crucial—it's the one chance to grab the attention of an admissions officer who may be reading thousands of essays. Personally, I also like to start out essays with an anecdote.

Strengths

The essay starts off strong. The story that the applicant shares in the first two paragraphs is interesting and personal. Her experience in public health is an asset to her application and she was wise to make it the theme of her essay. Her reasons for wanting to become an MD are clearly defined and her motivation is unquestioned. She effectively ties her conclusion to her introduction.

Weaknesses

The essay has some tense problems, particularly in the fourth paragraph. The transition from paragraph three to paragraph four is weak—it is almost redundant. It is the same case for the transition from paragraph four to five. The applicant probably felt that the subtle distinction in word choice made enough of a transition but the reality is that the introduction and conclusion to each paragraph is important and she did not make hers meaningful enough. The essay would have been much stronger had these issues been resolved.

ESSAY 20: Radiation Oncology Volunteer; Biochemical Lab Experience; Neurosurgery Research; ER Volunteer; English Language Tutor; Student Advisor; Community Service
Accepted at: Harvard Medical School

"Carl, the woman we're about to meet will receive her first palliative treatment today," said Dr. A., an Attending in Radiation Oncology. He continued to explain her case as we walked briskly down the hallways of the hospital. I followed him into the radiation treatment room to meet the patient and learn about the procedure which, sadly, would not eradicate her disease. Since then, I have met with him weekly throughout this summer to learn about radiation oncology and medicine in general. Through experiences such as these, I have learned much about the profession of medicine. I want to become a physician for the intellectual challenges and rewards that come from helping others.

I first became interested in medical research by working in a biochemical engineering laboratory at MIT. For over two years I explored the medically related field, biotechnology. I have led experiments involving fermentation bioreactors and trained two inexperienced undergraduates. Recently, I presented a poster entitled "Effect of Antifoam during Filtration of Recombinant Bacterial Broth" at a New England Society for Industrial Microbiology colloquium. Enjoying the biomedical rather than engineering aspects of the work, I have shifted my career interests to medicine.

Last summer, I expanded my interest in medicine by working for the Neurosurgery Department at Brigham and Women's Hospital. After a short training period, I worked independently on three research projects: Clonality analysis of schwannomas, clonality analysis of a multiple meningioma, and the loss of heterozygosity (LOH) screening of pituitary adenomas. I developed a strong interest in my work when I observed my mentor, Dr. Peter Black, remove brain tumors in the operating room. After the initial shock and amazement of seeing the exposed brain of a conscious patient, I thought more about the connections between this clinical work and my research. While my projects' objective was to gain a better understanding of tumors, the ultimate goal is to prevent and cure tumors to save human lives—the very people whom I had seen on the operating table! With this thought in mind, I found the motivation to complete the short-term objectives of my projects. I will be the second author of a paper, entitled "Clonality Analysis of Schwannomas," which will be submitted to Neurosurgery.

This summer, as a participant in NYU Medical Center's Summer Undergraduate Research Program (S.U.R.P.), I am learning even more about research and clinical medicine. In my work, I am determining the effect of the absence of the N-ras protooncogene on induced tumorigenesis. By conducting molecular oncology research for another summer, I have greatly expanded my knowledge and interest in the field. In addition, through my experiences in the Radiation Oncology Department with Dr. S., I clearly see the greater purpose of medical research beyond personal intellectual gratification. In the case of cancer and many other diseases, research is the only way to overcome the limitations of current clinical treatments.

I believe that one of the greatest joys and privileges of physicians are their abilities to directly aid and affect a community. While becoming interested in the science of medicine through research, I have explored human service to understand the art of medicine. When I volunteered in the Emergency Room of New England Medical Center during my sophomore year, many physicians impressed me with their sensitivity and compassion. When not assisting the hospital staff, I took every opportunity to comfort patients who felt scared and vulnerable. During that same year, I also tutored a middle-aged woman in English as a Second Language. It was challenging to teach her vocabulary and sentence structure since, initially, simple communication with her had been difficult. Helping her pass the high school equivalency exam made all of my efforts worthwhile. In addition, I have been an Associate Advisor for freshmen for the past two years. In this role, I have helped first year students adjust to college life. Not only have I played the role of academic mentor, but I have also become an intimate friend and personal tutor to my advisees. For my efforts, I won the annual Outstanding Associate Advisor Award.

Besides individual volunteering, I have taken the initiative to help the local community on a greater scale. As Community Service Chair for the Chinese Student's Club for the past two years, I established a new program to promote the interaction between MIT students and underprivileged teenagers. College students and children affiliated with a local community organization, Boston Asian: Youth Essential Service, have become acquainted through regular activities. Through the program, MIT volunteers help teenagers learn about the opportunities available at college. Along with several other undergraduates, I have become further acquainted with the teens through individual tutoring. To establish this new service program, I have done intensive planning and budget management. I have refined rough, creative ideas into organized activities involving over twenty people. During the planning stages, I have worked closely with professional youth counselors, other MIT participants, and the teens. While my involvement in this program has been very demanding at times, seeing these teens learn and develop their interests has definitely made it worthwhile.

During college I have learned many things outside of lecture halls and libraries. In research labs, I have refined my intellectual curiosity and scientific thought processes. In the local community, I have developed my interpersonal skills and a greater understanding of others. Through it all, I have learned to treasure the simple pleasures of helping others. By becoming a physician, I will continue to develop and apply these personal attributes.

Strengths

This is a solid essay that effectively communicates the applicant's motivation and reasons for wanting to attend medical school. Through the discussion of his research and volunteer experiences, he demonstrates that he has relevant experience, is qualified, and will likely succeed. The essay is well structured and easy to read.

Weaknesses

The essay is fairly standard. It won't jump out of the stack of essays as the most riveting or original but it serves the purpose adequately.

ESSAY 21: Late Interest in Medicine; Orphanage Volunteer in Brazil; Career Switcher from Consulting; Clinic Lab Assistant and History Taker

Accepted at: Stanford University School of Medicine; Harvard Medical School; Dartmouth Medical School; University of Massachusetts Medical School

When I entered Dartmouth College in 1987, I was amazed by the large number of students already labeled as "premeds." I wondered how those students were able to decide with such certainty that they wanted to study medicine, and I imagined that they all must have known from a very early age that they would one day be great doctors. I had no such inklings, and if asked as a child what I wanted to be when I grew up, I would have said that I wanted to be an Olympic skier or soccer player. While in high school, my achievement in various science courses prompted several friends and teachers to ask if I was interested in becoming a doctor. My negative response to their queries was largely based on my mistaken notion that since I didn't grow up knowing I wanted to be a doctor, I probably wasn't cut out for a career in medicine. I realize now that the decision to pursue a career in medicine must be based on much more than an instinctively positive feeling about becoming a doctor. I now know that making the decision to study medicine requires careful examination of one's reasons for wanting to be a doctor, an understanding of the rigors of medical training and the demanding nature of the profession, and perhaps most importantly, the maturity to make the great commitment that is necessary in order to achieve the goal of becoming an excellent physician.

People often ask me when I decided that I wanted to be a doctor. My response to that seemingly straight forward question is not a simple one since several years elapsed from the time that I initially became interested in medicine until I decided to apply to medical school. My job volunteering in an orphanage in Brazil during my sophomore year in college was extremely influential in shaping my current goals. At the orphanage, I lived with thirty young girls and four Portuguese-speaking, Japanese nuns in the countryside, several hours by car from Sao Paulo. My daily chores included everything from caring for babies and teaching the older girls English to harvesting vegetable crops before they were destroyed by summer floods and even fishing in the hopes of adding an extra source of protein to our diets. While helping out at the orphanage and getting to know the children was a unique and exciting experience, I was somewhat frustrated by the fact that I didn't have any specific skill or service to offer the people I met in Brazil. I considered what type of work I would like to do if I ever returned to Brazil or another developing country, and I began to think about how rewarding it would be to be a doctor in such a place where the need for even basic health care services was dire. Pursuing a career in medicine seemed like an ideal way to balance both my desire to work with disadvantaged people either abroad or at home and my desire to work in a dynamic, intellectually challenging field. However, I hesitated to commit myself to the difficult and time consuming goal of becoming a doctor, and I wondered whether my interest in medicine would endure when I returned to college or whether it was a transient manifestation of idealism engendered by my experience working with the poor in Brazil. As it turned out, thoughts of becoming a doctor never left me after living in Brazil, and although I didn't immediately commit myself to the idea of going to medical school, I decided to keep my options open by exploring some biology courses when I returned to Dartmouth.

I missed the sense of satisfaction that I had experienced while working with the children in Brazil when I began working for a management consulting firm after I graduated from college. Although I enjoyed the problem solving nature of consulting, my interest in improving the business practices of client companies was limited. I worked hard and performed well while in consulting, but I longed for a sense of accomplishment greater than that which I was able to realize while working in business. I began to consider returning to school to complete my medical school prerequisite courses, and I found that my perspective regarding the great commitment associated with a medical career had changed since college as a result of my experience working in business. I was excited rather than daunted when I thought about the challenges I would encounter in medical school and throughout my medical career because I had gained a new understanding of the importance of pursuing a career that I would find both intellectually stimulating and personally rewarding.

I returned to school after working in consulting for almost a year. While I enjoyed my pre-requisite science courses this past year, it was my experience volunteering as a patient history taker and a lab assistant at the Free Medical Clinic of Cleveland that truly confirmed my desire to be a doctor. As a history taker, I met with each patient before he or she was seen by a doctor, and I was responsible for recording each patient's relevant past history, current symptoms, and vital signs. Many of the people I interviewed were teenagers or young adults with health problems related to their sexual activity. After observing other history takers and conducting interviews myself, I gained confidence in my ability to ask pertinent questions based on preliminary information offered by the frequently scared or embarrassed patients, and I found that I was able to put patients at ease in situations that had the potential to be very uncomfortable for them. Working in the medical lab at the Clinic complemented my history taking experience. I observed which tests doctors ordered based on the different symptoms presented by patients,

I conducted some of the lab tests myself, and I observed the doctors interpret the test results that helped them make their diagnoses. I learned a great deal while working at the Clinic, and I left Cleveland feeling satisfied that I had contributed something to the community in which I had lived and looking forward to medical school more than ever.

My experiences taking pre-medical courses, volunteering at the Cleveland Free Clinic, and working with non-traditional, pre-medical students like myself at Harvard Summer School have all served to convince me that I want to be a practicing physician. I needed time after college to reach that conclusion, and I believe that I will be a better medical student, and hopefully a better doctor, as a result of my varied experiences and careful questioning of my motivations for wanting to become a doctor. I am currently anticipating the start of my new job working as a research assistant in the intensive care unit at Boston Children's Hospital, and I am confident that working at Children's Hospital will further strengthen my desire to pursue a career in medicine.

Student Comments

I worked hard on my essay to explain my decision to leave a job in consulting and to pursue a career in medicine. I think it's important for "nontraditional" applicants to give the chronology of the various things they have done, but more importantly to explain their motivation to leave behind other interesting opportunities and to accept the challenge of becoming a physician. Also, it is so important to be honest since one will be asked many times about the personal statement when interviewing, and it's painfully obvious when a student exaggerates or is overly dramatic when recounting their experiences (I served on the Harvard Medical School admissions committee).

Strengths

As a career-changing applicant, it was necessary to explain why he was motivated to return to college and complete premed courses and ultimately to apply to medical school. To that end, the applicant was on the right path.

Weaknesses

However, the length to which this topic was inefficiently discussed was exhausting. The applicant should have covered this topic more directly and in one paragraph. He should have used the remainder of the essay to discuss experiences that let the admissions committee get to know him better.

ESSAY 22: From a Family of Physicians; Late Interest in Medicine; Outward Bound Experience; Classics Major; Biomedical Lab Experience; Teaching Assistant
Accepted at: Harvard Medical School

One day in the summer after my graduation from high school, my grandfather took me up to the attic of his house to show me something he thought would be significant for me. He unwrapped a dusty silver bowl engraved with a barely legible inscription marking the graduation of my great-great grandfather from the University of South Carolina Medical School in 1837. My grandfather then proceeded to note that every W. male in a direct line down to me had chosen medicine as a career. The rather obvious hint was, of course, that he felt I should follow the same path; but it was at this moment that I decided a medical career would not be the definite goal during my four years in college. Indeed, I even resolved to investigate every possibility that interested me before I looked to medicine.

During that same summer, I placed my life in a real crucible during a three week Outward Bound trip in Utah. The incredible outdoor experience and the compelling philosophy of the Outward Bound School deeply affected my personality and my perceptions of my own life. I came to realize that the goals that I had previously held in such high esteem—success in terms of tangible criteria—now seemed less important; and I gained a much greater appreciation for the enjoyment of life by living on my own terms and being more completely aware of the environment and, especially, the people around me.

I thus entered Harvard that fall with optimism and a hunger to explore all of the possibilities which such an institution has to offer. I took no real science courses my freshman year in a conscious effort to explore new academic frontiers, and decided to major in the field that had always fascinated me—Classics. I soon found that I missed the sciences, however, and began to wonder if this was a sign that, despite my intentions, I would eventually be drawn back into the field I had consciously rejected.

After a summer working in a biomedical lab and two semesters of science during my sophomore year, my love of science had been rekindled, but I had not yet decided what path I would follow. I greatly enjoyed the Classics Department, but did not feel that I could study ancient texts for a lifetime. During the summer after my sophomore year, my appreciation for helping others which I had discovered two summers before in Utah led me to work as a teaching assistant at a summer school; and it was here that my mind was finally made up concerning my career plans. I enjoyed my teaching responsibilities, but it was my interaction with scores of new and interesting people at the school that really affected me. All of the students at the school were nearly my equals in age, yet they treated me with a respect and trust that I found extremely rewarding. I was there to help them grow and mature socially, as well as academically, and they placed complete confidence in me. To my delight, I was able to respond to this rather weighty responsibility and, I believe, help a few new friends hammer out their still-malleable personalities.

I received a great amount of joy from my summer school experience, and emerged from it with a newly focused career plan. When I stepped back to look at my life, I realized that my love of science could be coupled with the type of experience that I had that summer only in the medical profession. The respect and the ability to help fellow humans in their struggle to achieve happiness that are inherent in the medical profession are extremely attractive to me, and represent the overriding factors which have made me realize that medicine is the correct path for me which will lead to a rewarding, lifelong career.

Student Comments

I spent very little time on the essay (we had to turn it in to our premed advisor in April of our Junior Year, and I didn't revise it much afterwards)—several hours, max. I don't think it had a very great impact on my application—the interview is so much more important. I would advise people to just be honest in their essay and not try to say what they think people want to hear. If your essay doesn't jibe with your interview, it might hurt you.

Authors' Comments:

This essay does not have clear strengths and weaknesses; instead, it falls somewhere in the middle. A chronological thought process on how the applicant decided to become a doctor was a fine idea in theory. However, he failed to reveal any great epiphanies upon announcing his decision. It just boiled down to a fondness for science and a desire to help people, which are reasons that are given far too often in application essays. This essay would not stand out to an admissions committee, as it says nothing interesting or unique about the applicant. As the applicant states in his comments, the essay did not have a big impact on his application. Had his GPA and MCAT not been strong, this may not have been the case.

ESSAY 23: Pediatrics Volunteer; Toxicology Research Experience
Accepted at: Yale University School of Medicine; Dartmouth Medical School; Harvard Medical School

Every doctor remembers his first patient. Though I am not yet a physician, I will always remember my own first patient from my volunteer work in pediatrics at the Dartmouth-Hitchcock Medical Center. His name was J. He was born prematurely, and for most of his eight months, the hospital had been his home. I'll never forget how small and fragile he seemed as I held him. I rocked him gently, taking care not to disturb the jumbled array of tubes that overwhelmed his tiny body. At first, I was awkward and tentative, scared I might in some way hurt this little baby. With time, however, I relaxed and was able to coax a smile out of him. What struck me most about J. was that, in spite of everything, he never once cried. From the feeding tube to the unfamiliar hands that cradled him, nothing fazed him.

In the following weeks, I became very involved in J.'s case. I learned to feed and change him, I walked with him around the ward, and a bond developed between us. One week, I arrived at the hospital to find a flurry of activity in J.'s room. I was overjoyed to discover that, at long last, he was healthy enough to leave the hospital! Weeks later, I inquired about J.'s progress, and was devastated to learn he had died at home. Tears welled in my eyes as I remembered the little baby who never cried.

Though my time with J. was short, our relationship has had a long-lasting effect on me. The experience confirmed my interest in pediatric medicine. I have worked with many patients in the three years since J., but he stands out in my mind. He taught me the true meaning of Sir William Osler's words: "The practice of medicine calls equally for the exercise of the heart and the head."

Volunteering has become a permanent part of my jam-packed college schedule. I get as much out of my weekly visits to the pediatrics ward as the children do. At the end of a hectic week, I look forward to sitting on the playroom floor, attempting some new activity with the youngsters. I've worked with everything from papier maché to popsicle sticks. Even though my inventive projects don't always result in the most successful artistic creations, the kids still enjoy them. They still smile, laugh, and have fun, like all children do.

After three years, I've become a familiar face on the fifth floor. I'm not the only permanent fixture, though. Week after week, I see many of the same youngsters and their families. As a result of cancer, the hospital has become part of their lives. I'm always amazed by the resilience of these children. More so than adults, they seem able to accept illness and adapt to the toll that treatment imposes on their lives. What strikes me most is the openness and honesty with which they speak about a subject that makes most adults uncomfortable. Hearing the medical terms roll off their tongues, it's easy to forget just how young these patients are. Only when they switch to talking about Nintendo or the latest Disney movie is one reminded they're still kids. Cancer doesn't change that.

My volunteer work provided the initial impetus behind my current involvement in cancer research. Having seen the effects of cancer on the human body, I became interested in learning about the molecular mechanisms behind the disease. For the past year, I have been working in the Department of Pharmacology and Toxicology at Dartmouth Medical School. The focus of my particular research project has been mitomycin C, a genotoxic carcinogen which induces DNA crosslinks. Last fall, I was awarded a Howard Hughes Biological Sciences Internship to investigate the effects of this drug on the expression of a hormone-inducible gene in the chick embryo. What began as a leave term project has evolved into an intensive, ongoing study which will culminate this spring in a senior honors thesis.

In an essay from The Fragile Species, Lewis Thomas notes that "Most of the investigators, the young ones especially, have only a remote idea of the connection of their work to human disease problems. . ." Through my research experience and my volunteer work, I have learned this connection. I often think of my young friends from the hospital when working in the laboratory. They provide the motivation that keeps me moving ahead with the next experiment. . . when the last one failed.

Strengths

This is a very strong essay. It is moving, personal, and effective at selling the applicant as a motivated and qualified candidate. Her relevant experience is offered through heart-wrenching stories in the pediatric ward and her impressive research is seamlessly tied into this theme. The applicant makes a huge impact in few words.

Weaknesses

None.

ESSAY 24: From a Family of Physicians; Motivated since Childhood; ER Volunteer; Chemistry Tutor and Teaching Assistant; Inorganic Chemistry and Molecular Biology Lab Experience
Accepted at: Harvard Medical School; University of Illinois College of Medicine

Initially, my interest in medicine was due to my family. Several of my relatives are physicians and they have always been enthusiastic about their hospital work. From their discussions on various diseases, I became very curious and disturbed about why all human beings inevitably age and die. I grew up being both impressed with all of the medical treatments available and dismayed by stories of the terminally ill. The human body was repairable but fragile. To be alive and healthy was a fascination.

These childhood impressions were strong ones, and when I began college, I felt deeply intrigued with medicine. During my college years, I studied a good deal of chemistry and biology, and as my interests in various sciences grew, I tried some hospital volunteer work. While pursuing my assorted interests, my captivation with medicine not only endured, but has remained to be my ultimate interest.

My most direct exposure to medicine was my volunteer work in hospital emergency rooms. The most enjoyable part of my job was taking patients who were on stretchers or in wheelchairs to various areas of the hospital and keeping them company. I enjoyed doing so, and I also found myself wishing that I had the skill and knowledge to examine and treat them. I also noticed how the physicians, nurses and aides all worked together. I was left with a vivid impression that the hospital was a close-knit team of different professionals, of which I wished to be a part of.

Teaching chemistry has also been a very positive experience. During my sophomore year and junior years, I was a tutor for an accelerated chemistry lab course. Acting on the belief that more help should be available for this rigorous class, I began a tutoring program, which continues to this day. I could relate to the students frustrations and I held classroom sessions for groups of students ranging from 5 to 25, covering questions dealing with laboratory procedures, reports and problem sets. After two years of tutoring, I felt it would be more challenging to teach a different class and I am presently a teaching assistant for a chemistry lecture course. From these teaching experiences, I have learned to communicate effectively to large groups of people and also to individuals on a one-to-one basis. I have become more sensitive to people's problems and needs and create an environment that encourages discussions and questions. My relationships with the students has been the most gratifying aspect of teaching, and as a physician, I hope to feel the same type of satisfaction from interacting with my patients.

During my summers, I have had an opportunity to work in various research laboratories. In order to sample different areas in science, I worked in labs ranging from inorganic chemistry to molecular biology. In all cases, I learned to conduct experiments in an orderly yet creative manner and I was constantly collecting data and interpreting results. Most importantly, I learned to accept my defeats graciously when my experiments failed. Last summer at MIT, I performed many experiments with unsatisfactory results, but I was able to finish my project and I will be the first author of a publication.

By becoming a physician, I will be able to solve medical problems while treating and being in constant contact with patients. Being a physician will be quite demanding and difficult at times, but most of all, I imagine that it will be most enjoyable and quite satisfying.

Student Comments

In my essay, I just wrote about things I felt proud of: my family background, volunteer work, teaching and research. I could have written much more on my research experience but I didn't because I knew that my recommendation letters would include that information in detail.

In terms of medical school admission advice, I tell people that just like in real life, connections are very important and so the letters of recommendation are very crucial. Yes, I had all A's and my MCAT scores were good but I think my letters of recommendation were almost the most important. Many students at Harvard (my classmates right now) also took an extra year to do research work and that also helps greatly in terms of a strong recommendation letter and what kind of an essay you can write by taking extra time off to do research and volunteer work. It is also very much worth the experience.

Strengths

The essay is well structured and has a nice progression from the applicant's first inspiration to pursue medicine, to relevant coursework, to volunteer work and teaching, and finally research. Most elements of an aptly written personal statement are here.

Weaknesses

The essay lacks punch and personality. It is not personal and it tells no interesting stories that allow the applicant to stand out to the admissions committee. It is a standard application essay written by a qualified candidate.

ESSAY 25: Ph.D. Candidate in Human Genetics Research; Cold Fusion Lab Experience; Technical Background; Computational Biology Lab Experience
Accepted at: Harvard Medical School; MIT Division of Health Sciences and Technology Program

I am interested in participating in the Harvard MIT Division of Health Sciences and Technology Program (HST) in the context of an M.D./Ph.D.

to prepare for a career in medical research. The knowledge of human biology and disease afforded by an M.D. program, particularly with the analytical focus of HST, will allow me to conduct more applied, medically relevant research in human genetics than Ph.D. training alone. I believe my computational background makes me a strong applicant for HST.

I majored in Physics at Dartmouth because the analytical and problem-solving aspects of the discipline appealed to me. During my sophomore year, I participated in the Science and Engineering Research Semester program at Los Alamos National Laboratory, sponsored by the Department of Energy. My work there, which involved data entry and analysis for cold fusion experiments, increased my familiarity with computer programming and graphics and enhanced my understanding of nuclear fusion. Furthermore, it exposed me to the systematic problem-solving approach used by research physicists in attacking a problem. I was stimulated by the research atmosphere at Los Alamos and excited by the prospect of a career in scientific research. However, I was disenchanted with the possible social and military applications of physics research.

I became interested in biology because of its potential for research of more direct social value. During my junior summer, I participated in the Undergradate Research Program at Cold Spring Harbor Laboratory, sponsored by the National Science Foundation. I worked in the lab of Dr. T., a computational biologist, and returned to his lab after graduation as a permanent employee. My work at Cold Spring Harbor has been part of a project to create a database of "Short Functional Elements" of DNA and protein. Recently I have been investigating the role of a specific seven-amino acid signal with a particularly interesting pattern of distribution, including p53 tumor suppressor and several families of tyrosine kinases. My work involves writing and using computer programs for sequence analysis, reading technical papers, and conferring with other scientists at the lab. I truly enjoy my research at the lab because of the academic nature of the work and the social and medical implications of studying signal transduction in the cell. In addition, this experience has advanced my undergraduate computational training and expanded my knowledge of molecular and cell biology and genetics.

I have developed a strong interest in pursuing a career in biology research as a result of my experience at Cold Spring Harbor. I am particularly interested in the field of human genetics, and feel that combined M.D./Ph.D. training with the particular quantitative emphasis of HST will best prepare me to conduct competitive research with socially meaningful applications.

Strengths

Although this is a very straightforward, albeit dry essay, it effectively answers the question of why the applicant wishes to pursue the MD/PhD program. Through the discussion of his research and undergraduate focus, the applicant comes across as very intelligent and competent. Because his career goal is research based and not patient care, the direct and nonpersonal style of his essay is almost fitting.

Weaknesses

The essay has no real weaknesses. If his goals were patient care, showing more of his personality through his experiences would be recommended.

ESSAY 26: Cold Fusion Lab Experience; Fellowship for After-school Literacy Program; Computational Biology Lab Experience
Accepted at: Yale University School of Medicine; University of Pennsylvania School of Medicine; Johns Hopkins University School of Medicine; New York University School of Medicine

I am interested in pursuing an M.D. degree as part of a combined M.D.-Ph.D. program because I feel that this course of study will best prepare me for competitive research in human genetics. A Ph.D. program will help me develop strong research skills, and a degree in medicine will provide me with knowledge of human biology and medicine from a less abstract, more "human" perspective that will allow me to conduct research of direct social and medical value. My academic background and research experience have adequately prepared me to complete such a demanding course of graduate study.

During my sophomore year, I participated in the Science and Engineering Research Semester program at Los Alamos National Laboratory, sponsored by the Department of Energy. I was incredibly stimulated by the research atmosphere and the academic challenge of the work. The environment which surrounded and supported the research at Los Alamos encouraged discussion and endless questioning. My work there, which involved data entry and analysis for cold fusion experiments, increased my familiarity with computer programming and graphics and enhanced my understanding of nuclear fusion. Furthermore, it exposed me to the systematic problem-solving approach used by research physicists in attacking a problem. While I was excited by the prospect of a career in scientific research, however, I was disenchanted with the possible social and military applications of physics research.

My reactions to this experience were reaffirmed during the following fall when I received a fellowship from Dartmouth's Tucker Foundation to work for the Center for Family Life in Brooklyn, New York, devising and implementing an after-school literacy program in which junior high school students tutored elementary school children. This job was the perfect complement to my term at Los Alamos. The fulfillment I experienced working in Brooklyn reinforced my desire for socially meaningful and constructive work, while the lack of an intense academic atmosphere was ultimately unsatisfying.

During the following summer, I participated in the Undergradate Research Program at Cold Spring Harbor Laboratory, sponsored by the National Science Foundation. I worked in the lab of Dr. T., a computational biologist, and returned to his lab after graduation as a permanent employee. My work at Cold Spring Harbor has been part of a project to create a database of "Short Functional Elements" of DNA and protein. Recently I have been investigating the role of a specific seven-amino acid signal with a particularly interesting pattern of distribution, including p53 tumor suppressor and several families of tyrosine kinases. My work involves writing and using computer programs for sequence analysis, reading technical papers, and conferring with other scientists at the lab.

Working at Cold Spring Harbor has been rewarding for a number of reasons. Most importantly, I truly enjoy my research because of the academic nature of the work and of the atmosphere at the lab in general, and because of the social and medical implications of studying signal transduction in the cell. This project has also advanced my undergraduate computational training and expanded my knowledge of molecular and cell biology and genetics. Finally, I have been fortunate enough to attend many meetings, lectures and conferences held at the lab, including the 40th anniversary of Watson and Crick's discovery of the double helix structure of DNA. Participating in that celebration was a privilege for me and strongly reinforced my desire to work in a research environment and conduct research as a career.

Each of these experiences has helped me evaluate what is important to me in choosing a career. I believe an M.D.-Ph.D. degree will best enable me to achieve my goals of becoming a successful researcher and performing socially meaningful work.

The same applicant who wrote Essay 25 wrote this essay but it was submitted to different schools. The essays are very similar and our feedback on each is consistent.

Strengths

This is a well-constructed, straightforward essay that effectively expresses the applicant's motivation for an MD/PhD program. Although it is not very personal, it is interesting enough to hold the attention of the reader. It successfully convinces the reader that the applicant is intelligent and qualified and a career in research seems fitting.

Weaknesses

The essay has no personality and we do not get to know much about the applicant through his words. Although the essay may have been more interesting had it been more personal, its no-nonsense style seems suitable from an applicant pursuing a career in research.

ESSAY 27: Childhood Car Accident; Soup Kitchen and ER Volunteer and Big Sister; Biomedical Research Experience; Competitive Tennis

Accepted at: Harvard Medical School; Ohio State University College of Medicine; University of Pittsburgh School of Medicine; Albert Einstein College of Medicine, Yeshiva University

The car swerved to the left. A sudden impact forced me out of my sitting position in the back of the station wagon. Everything became still as I heard the uneasy voice of my mother's friend in the driver's seat: "Mrs. K., Mrs. K.!" She became frantic and started crying, muttering phrases that I did not understand. What I did know was that my mother was not answering her cries. I sat and stared at the back of the passenger's seat of the car, trying to make sense of what was happening. I was seven and the only thing I knew was that something was wrong. I did not cry, I did not call out to my mom. I sat frozen, listening intently for my mother's voice, watching my mom's friend plead through tears, and wondering why she was not doing anything to help her. A short while later, ambulances arrived. After someone helped me out of the car, I tried to get to my mom. The paramedics would not let me near her, but I saw her with her head tilted back into the seat and groaning softly. Her eyelids were shut but the shape and wrinkles of her face told me that she was in immense pain.

My mother broke her right arm in the accident, leaving her unable to care for my seven-month-old sister. At first seeing my mother so helpless was as distressing as my fear during the accident. During the next several months, I discovered that the act of helping allayed my fears. Even now my mother's face glows with affection each time she recalls how at the age of seven, I helped bathe, feed, and change the diapers of my baby sister. The desire to help care for my mom and my sister was instinctive; she never needed to ask.

Driven by this instinct, the urge to learn through helping has remained strong. In high school I helped cook and serve meals in a soup kitchen on Sundays. I also devoted my time to the E.R. of Lake West Hospital. Upon graduating, I worked in the pediatric I.C.U. of the Cleveland Clinic. Since then, I have also volunteered at the Massachusetts General Hospital. All of these opportunities have been invaluable, but the most rewarding has been my role as a Big Sister for an eight-year-old girl through the United Way Big Sister Association. Y. emigrated with her family from Hong Kong only one year ago. Her family, lacking both the financial resources and the knowledge of English, is rarely able to take her out of Chinatown and introduce her to her new environment. In spite of our language barrier, Y. and I have become fast friends through six hour outings every Saturday. From patiently teaching her "Mary Had a Little Lamb" on the piano to drawing pictures to explain why "my daddy and mommy" do not live in my dorm room, I truly enjoy every moment with her. What makes this volunteer job so much more meaningful than the others is that it does not end at the end of my shift. It means I can come back to my dorm room after a tiring day of classes, play back my answering machine, and hear her sweet voice sing a Chinese lullaby for me. It means that this is not a volunteer job: She gives just as much to me as I give to her.

My eagerness to care for others coupled with my father's influence as a physician developed my interest in health care through biomedical research. Specifically, I have worked independently on two projects. I mastered cell culture techniques to study the effects of nerve and epidermal growth factors on amyloid precursor protein ectodomain secretion in rat pheochromocytoma cells (applied to Alzheimer's disease). I was fortunate enough to obtain favorable results which are in the process of being published. My current project is analyzing the effects of leptin, the protein product of the obesity gene, on insulin regulation (applied to diabetes). I am responsible for conducting and quantifying experiments in pancreatic beta cell lines, as well as assaying insulin, corticosteroid, and glucose levels of experiments done in vivo. My enjoyment of laboratory research stems from two levels. First, being directly involved in the process of uncovering new knowledge, rather than simply absorbing knowledge uncovered by others is exhilarating. Second, the road of many hours of hard work and repetition resolving in a slow but stimulating process is familiar and encouraging—I have traveled this same road by playing ten years of competitive tennis.

I realize that succeeding in medicine requires more than a desire to help others. A career in medicine demands great perseverance and dedication to both scientific and humanistic knowledge. I believe I have acquired these characteristics through my academic, extracurricular, and research experiences. These qualities in addition to my concern for others will enable me to care for my future patients with sensitivity and understanding. The once bewildered seven-year-old at the scene of an accident now has the skills and maturity to do more than change diapers; she aspires to read the film of the broken humerus or to set the cast some day soon.

Student Comments

My advice would be to try to include things that do NOT show up elsewhere on your application that you feel might be relevant. When starting out, make a list of jobs/personal qualities/events that you would like to include and among those, see if you can connect them into a "theme" for your essay.

Strengths

This is an interesting essay because it begins with a personal story that gives the reader insight into the applicant's life as a child and into experiences that have motivated who she is today. It is well structured—ending with a conclusion that ties into the story she shares in the opening. She seized the opportunity to highlight soft qualities that were not found elsewhere in her application.

Weaknesses

While the opening story was engaging, and adequately covers the topic of motivation, succinctly presenting it in one paragraph instead of two would have left space for experiences that showcase more of the applicant's skills and qualities.

ESSAY 28: Art History Major; Peer Educator; Au Pair in Iceland; Hospital Intern in Paris; Fulbright Scholar

Accepted at: University of California—San Francisco School of Medicine; Johns Hopkins University School of Medicine; Stanford University School of Medicine; Cornell University Medical College; University of Pennsylvania School of Medicine; Columbia University College of Physicians and Surgeons; Yale University School of Medicine; University of Virginia School of Medicine; Harvard Medical School; Washington University School of Medicine

When I consider my life experiences, I imagine them as a system of bones and joints, interconnected, cooperative, and form-giving. Much as a living organism is built on its skeletal network, I have arisen from a body of connections that provides structure to my life and a foundation for continued growth. Since I was very young, I have searched for links between people, places, and academic disciplines, both to broaden my appreciation of them and to demonstrate the merits of human interaction and cooperation.

In my high school advanced placement course in biology, I was fascinated by our dissection of a fetal pig, for it satisfied both my scientific and my artistic curiosity. On that day I was both surgeon and sculptor, and my growing interest in the field of medicine was confirmed by this simple demonstration of the union of two disciplines. Now, as an undergraduate pre-medical candidate majoring in art history, having recently written my senior thesis on the science of seventeenth- and eighteenth-century French painting, I have confirmed for myself that in every academic discipline there are elements of others and that any research endeavor offers the possibility for new connections within the wide panorama of intellectual perspectives.

Through my experiences on varsity team sports and as a health educator, for example, I have come to appreciate human cooperation as a basis for individual strength. To be successful, a team must be flexible, cohesive, and aware that it is only as strong as its weakest player. These lessons on the playing field demonstrate to me the value of communication in all areas of human interaction. As a peer educator for the Princeton Health Center, I serve both as advisor and listener in the exchange of ideas. This role not only confirms for me the value of interpersonal relations; it provides me with confidence in myself to educate others on important health issues.

Finally my experiences as an au pair in Iceland, as an exchange student in Lyons, France, and as an intern at a hospital in Paris, France, have taught me the importance of international exchange and communication. These opportunities abroad provided me with complete immersion in a foreign language and culture, practice in adaptability, and an expanding vision of the benefits of cross-cultural connections. I am convinced that my study in Oxford next year as a Fulbright scholar will heighten my enthusiasm for international cooperation in efforts to advance medical research. My work in glycobiology will not only allow me to link current biomedical developments to this emerging field; it will provide me with the opportunity to bridge distant cultures in the pursuit of collective human understanding and achievement.

My search for connections is not over. Just as I envisage the world as a network of interrelated people, ideas, and goals, so I see myself as a microcosm of this system in which each experience both connects to and supports every other. With such a stable yet developing foundation, I am eager to add flesh to the skeleton in medical school.

Strengths

The applicant demonstrates that she is well rounded and bright. She includes many experiences that may not be found elsewhere on her application.

Weaknesses

The essay lacks personality. It reads like a list of experiences that the applicant jotted down before starting the essay. None of the experiences were discussed with enough substance to make them interesting or personal. The analogy of her life experiences to a skeletal network, which is a reference made over and over, was an attempt at creative writing that did not effectively enhance her essay.

ESSAY 29: Father's Influence; Motivation Since Childhood; Hospital Lab Assistant; Biology M.S.; Cloning Research Experience; Teaching Assistant
Accepted at: Harvard Medical School

My father's greatest impact on me occurred in the form of a story taken from the Hindu epic Mahabharta about Arjuna, the great Indian archer who, when aiming his arrow, would see only the center of the target and would be rendered oblivious to his surroundings. Each of my pursuits ultimately inspires this kind of passion and single-minded dedication. While I have wanted to become a physician ever since I was a child, medicine did not engender such commitment until four years ago when I worked as a hospital lab assistant. That summer was the first time I came face to face with my dreams. Youthful idealism gave way to reality as I worked directly with patients and physicians and I learned how to draw blood, obtain throat cultures, and prepare stool and urine samples for analysis. But I discovered that medicine involved more than these skills, for my work introduced me to an array of emotions that seemed to lie at the heart of medicine. There were humorous moments—a woman once thanked me repeatedly after learning of her positive pregnancy test and I responded by assuring her that I had nothing to do with it. There were also painful moments, such as when I drew blood from George, a 97-year-old man dying of cancer. Suddenly, I became interested in the lives of patients I encountered sometimes only for a few minutes each day. I enjoyed the intermingling of emotions that occurred at patients bedsides with the scientific analysis that occurred in the lab. Becoming a physician was no longer a dream—it was a goal I was determined to achieve.

However, my desire to treat patients is only part of my motivation to study medicine. During my sophomore year, an introductory biology

146

class instilled in me a fascination with molecular biology experimental techniques and their usefulness in discovering the causes of human diseases. I was intrigued by the notion that microscopic problems such as viral infections could lead to macroscopic problems such as leukemia and hepatitis—the same diseases I had encountered at the hospital. I decided to major in biology but, wanting to study the field in depth, I entered Stanford's coterminal program, allowing me to pursue B.S. and M.S. degrees in biology simultaneously.

A year later, my molecular biology interest motivated me to work with Dr. I. on a research project cloning the gene for an integrin which directs lymphocytes to inflammatory sites and obtaining antibodies against the integrin. Understanding these antibodies structures might allow the production of treatments for inflammatory diseases like arthritis. While these long-term clinical applications initially attracted me to the project, I discovered that research also offered the more immediate satisfaction of working independently and systematically dissecting each facet of a scientific problem in search of an answer. The pleasure I derived from research offered a striking contrast to the interactions with people and opportunity to help people that made my hospital job rewarding. I also learned that satisfaction in research doesn't just come from success for, even when I failed, each failure increased my understanding of the techniques and brought me closer to success.

Having encountered the various facets of learning as an aspiring medical scientist, I grew interested in teaching and became one of the few undergraduates ever appointed teaching assistant for the third course in Stanford's biology core. My job was to grade exams and lead two weekly discussion sections of twenty students each. However, cognizant of each student's potential and the benefits they would derive from greater commitment on my part, I prepared handouts containing extra problems, held office hours to further assist students, and encouraged students to probe beyond the classroom level. The satisfaction of seeing understanding register in student's faces and fostering their budding interest in the material was well worth my efforts.

After witnessing the limits of existing medical technology in a hospital and feeling the gratification of trying to overcome these limits through research, my initial interest in treating the sick has evolved into a desire to discover innovative treatments in the laboratory and implement them at the bedside. Because I have had clinical experiences in which I directly administered patient care and research experiences in which I followed my own projects from start to finish, I know that an academic medicine career would be satisfying. I aspire to be a medical school professor—as a researcher, I would gather knowledge; as a physician, I would use this knowledge to heal; and, as a teacher, I would disseminate this knowledge to future physicians.

Strengths

The applicant demonstrates a commitment to the field through his hospital and research experience.

Weaknesses

The applicant has poor writing skills as evidenced by his grammatical errors. His lack of correct punctuation made the essay awkward and difficult to read. The opening line was never effectively incorporated into the essay and his father's impact, although mentioned, was never explained. Although there was some substance to the essay, it was weak overall due to the applicant's lack of solid writing skills.

ESSAY 30: Archaeology Thesis Analyzing Bones of Prehistoric Woman
Accepted at: Harvard Medical School

As part of my senior thesis, I learned the remarkable story of a woman. I learned her story not through words but through her bones. My thesis consisted of cataloging, collecting data and analyzing a skeletal collection, consisting of this woman and approximately twenty-five other Chugach Eskimo excavated in the 1930's. They were to be reburied as part of the mandated repatriation of Native American remains. I volunteered to catalog the collection by myself to gather data for my senior thesis. These data now serve as the permanent record for the collection at the University Museum of Archaeology and Anthropology at the University of Pennsylvania.

This woman, known simply to me as Palutat Cave B-1, gradually unfolded to me the extraordinary story of her life by letting what remained of her body speak for her. She was a battered woman. Her bones bore the marks traditionally associated with battering. She had three healed wounds in the back of the skull, believed to be the result of her attempts to escape her batterer only to be struck in the head from behind. From X-ray films, it was learned that her left forearm had also been broken (parry fracture) as she attempted to ward off blows. It is very possible that she was battered much more often than her wounds indicate. Clearly only a small fraction of blows are strong enough to leave their mark on the skeleton. At some point, infection entered the wounds to her left forearm, and osteomyelitis set in. The osteomyelitis became severe and spread to her wrist and elbow. Somehow, she managed to live for at least another year. Eventually there was complete ankylosis of the carpals, and virtually all cortical bone in the radius and ulna was lost.

Thus her forearm was rendered dysfunctional. During that time, her left humerus and scapula underwent substantial disuse atrophy, a clear indication that the arm was of no use to her. Instead she used her teeth to hold objects and assist in the performance of daily tasks, as shown by the greatly increased amount of wear on her incisors. Yet somehow, she managed to live to the age where the protein-rich diet of the Chugach takes it toll in the form of osteoporosis. Probably unrelated to previous trauma, her T12 vertebra had collapsed. Although aging an archeological sample is more art than science, she most likely died in her thirties.

After sixty years in the University Museum, Palutat Cave B-1 is now at home and at peace in Prince William Sound, Alaska, in a cedar coffin made by her descendants. I am grateful for the extraordinary opportunity I had to learn part of her story. Although it is difficult to speculate about temperament or attitude, this woman must have been strong and determined to have survived as long as she did. Her life was clearly filled with physical pain. As I put together her story, I began to feel for this woman who had struggled so hard to survive. It was a strange feeling to be able to piece together this woman's story of pain by the scars it had left on her bones. I felt both impressed by this woman who had survived so much and excited for having been able to extract so much information from bones alone. I had enjoyed it, but in the end, I could do nothing to help her. My experience with Palutat Cave B-1 and the rest of the Chugach collection has given me a great respect for the ability of the human body to adapt to adversity. I saw firsthand the results of the skeletal system's response to stressful conditions: trauma, disease, and inadequate nutrition. I am still amazed at the efficiency of the skeletal system and its incredible ability to deal with adverse conditions.

To a large extent, my choice to become a physician is rooted in my desire to continue to work with the human body. But I want to work with the living. I want to work with people I can help. As a physician, I will be able to assist the human body in the healing process. Though my work with the Chugach collection inspired me to learn more about the human body, it lacked the element of genuine human interaction. This is a feature of medicine I have found to be especially appealing in my experience since graduating from Penn. I want to continue to learn and to discover more about the human body through work with people and through the study of medicine.

Student Comments

I wrote this after graduating from Penn. I did not complete any of my pre-med courses while in college, and returned to do the Post-Bac Premed program at Penn. The Director of the PBPM program at Penn kept a copy of this essay to give to future students.

Strengths

This is a unique essay that will certainly stand out to the admissions committee. It tells a story within a story. As the applicant reveals her experience in anthropology, she also tells an engaging story of the life of one of her research subjects. It was a cleverly crafted essay that will give the admissions committee a nice break from the monotony of the standard application essay. Through the description of her work experience, she effectively communicates her inspiration to study medicine.

Weaknesses

None.

ESSAY 31: Worked on Grandfather's Farm in Hungary; Orderly/ Surgery Assistant in Former U.S.S.R.; Organized Financing for First Private Hospital in Estonia and Mission for Bosnian Refugees

Accepted at: Harvard Medical School

In communist Hungary in 1986 ownership of property meant certain things. It meant that you were envied by your neighbors. It meant that you were mistrusted by the state. It meant that you were prohibited by a government which feared the reemergence of a landed aristocracy from purchasing machinery or hiring laborers. Above all it meant you held on to your land for all you were worth and cherished it as your most precious family heirloom.

In 1986 and in the following summer, my parents sent my sister and I to Hungary to work on my Grandparent's farm as they were getting old and unable to manage it any longer on their own, particularly in light of the communist restrictions on private landowners. I woke up at five, harvested hay by hand, tended the cows, and spread manure. I used the same tools my great-grandfather used and on the same land that he had tended a century ago. A fifteen year old boy with little sense of responsibility or of himself, the experience hit me with the force of a cyclone.

In 1993 I was awarded a fellowship to work in the health sector of the former Estonian Republic of the U.S.S.R. I was employed as an orderly in the operating theater of what was once the elite Communist Party hospital. I assisted in surgery, performed twenty-four hour shifts, distributed humanitarian aid, and wrote reports for the Ministry of Health that went from my hands to the directors of the World Bank and U.N. World Health Organization. The experience cemented my plans for becoming a physician and also convinced me that I wanted a career with policy- and theory-shaping responsibilities beyond those of the ordinary doctor.

In addition to being entrusted with work no twenty-one year old in America would be allowed to perform. I saw history being written before my eyes. I got a sense of the degree to which an individual, with enough motivation and a few good ideas, can be an effective force for positive change. I understood the responsibility and the capacity we all have to work for the good of society. The experience was tremendously empowering as it gave me the perspective and self confidence to attempt to seize the future and the ambition to attempt to change the world to the degree I can. With two other Columbia students and a group of Estonian doctors I organized an attempt to finance the first private hospital in Estonia which indirectly contributed to the first Estonian laws on health care privatization and reform. Since my return I have with another Columbia student organized a mission to travel to the N. camp in southern Hungary to distribute clothing and medical supplies to the Bosnian refugees. My role has been in the obtaining of funds and in acting as an intermediary between our group of 10 Columbia University students, two of whom spent this past summer working in the camp, and Hungarian officials here and in Hungary.

I became an adult during my first summer in Hungary. The same changes that have allowed my grandfather to hold onto his land allowed me to first test in Estonia the wings I had developed years earlier. I hope to use those wings make an impact on medical science. Genetics and biochemistry represent the future of medicine and the area in which someone with ambition, a desire to work for the public good, and the necessary technical background could make the most significant contribution. Motivation, independence, maturity, precisely those qualities my experiences in Eastern Europe instilled, will be essential to a fruitful career. I can imagine none potentially more fulfilling, nor a more worthy aim for my life's work, than connecting the worlds of medical science and international public health.

Strengths

The applicant shares some very unique and interesting experiences that will allow him to stand out to the admissions committee. His experiences also reveal a competent, hard-working, and caring individual. The essay begins very strong, sparking immediate interest from the reader. His motivation to pursue a career in medicine, along with his commitment to the field, is effectively communicated.

Weaknesses

There are no weaknesses in terms of content. The essay had some typos and grammatical errors, particularly with punctuation. If the applicant had sought a grammatical review, the essay would have been even stronger.

ESSAY 32: Classical Musician; Career Switch from Music and Psychology; Teacher in Indonesia; Author; Psychobiological Research
Accepted at: Harvard Medical School

The melody starts low, a quiet whirring sound of violins slowly envelops the hall. The audience is quiet, hushed; the rustling of programs, coughs and seat adjustments stilled. The initial theme is laid out like a red velvet blanket. Another theme then appears, complementing the first, yet affirming its own identity with each new twist of the melody.

The evolution of my life, from classical musician to research psychologist to pre-medical student can be likened to the thematic development in a symphony. I grew up with a younger sister who was profoundly retarded, and learned the rewards that come with putting one's own problems aside and doing something for others. This guided my initial interests in psychology and also in music, as she and her schoolmates often responded enthusiastically to my guitar playing and singing. In my early twenties, five years living in Paris were like a modulation into a new key or tonality: The elements from the initial melody were still recognizable, but the new setting allowed a different set of colors to emerge. I learned about discipline, hard work, patience, and humility through both successes and disappointments while learning to sing opera, operetta, and lieder in France. I also explored the therapeutic applications of music by assisting a deaf musical therapist, and occasionally volunteering at a school for the deaf in Paris. I came to Boston five years later, fluent in French, to continue music at the New England Conservatory of Music. While at the conservatory, I co-founded and co-supervised a community outreach program, in which students volunteered to perform in local nursing homes, hospices, homeless shelters, and prisons.

After completing the Conservatory, I had the opportunity to teach music and sing in Indonesia. During this brief time, I was struck with the remarkable ability of economically disadvantaged children to find hope and beauty in the face of poverty and hardship. I became intrigued with the concept of resiliency, and on returning to Boston, began working with researchers on the psychobiological effects of trauma. This eventually led to a Master's degree in Psychology from Harvard University, ten co-authored publications and book chapters, and academic appointments at Harvard

Medical School and at Massachusetts General Hospital. During this time, I thanked the years of musical training in voice, piano, and French horn that enabled me to work and learn in unsupervised environments and to persevere over complex problems with a focused concentration.

Tonality is a function of the fundamental tone: Everything that makes up tonality emanates from that tone and refers back to it. But even though it refers back, that which emanates has a life of its own; it is independent. While working at the hospital, I was promoted to Research Coordinator, and ran several different psychobiological studies. One project that I found particularly intriguing was investigating the psychophysiological manifestations of traumatic hyperarousal in Posttraumatic Stress Disorder patients. At this point, I realized that clinical research and science were fulfilling in a way that music never had been. Working with a team to develop theories that could then be applied to alleviate emotional and physical distress seemed to be the best use of my intellectual and creative abilities. I began to think about a career in medicine with a certainty that has since crescendoed from a pianissimo to a resounding forte. Other crystallizing experiences in my decision-making process include working under the auspices of the Albert Schweitzer Organization, using my skills learned at the Trauma Clinic to train mental health clinicians from the former Yugoslavia.

Whether writing up the results of clinical research or preparing an operatic role, a certain amount of creativity is involved. However, inspiration does not replace a solid technique nor a thorough knowledge base. My interest in studying medicine is to gain a comprehensive understanding of the human system and its pathologies, both physical as well as psychological. I have been inspired by the physicians with whom I have worked, particularly the importance they place on careful observation in their clinical work, and their willingness to sacrifice pet theories in favor of the truth. Working closely with them has heightened my zeal for doing medicine and has contributed to my dedication to apply science in a meaningful way.

Learning to listen to oneself is a trait that most musicians spend their entire lives attempting to acquire. The experiences that I have had in thirty years have led me to a greater, albeit imperfect, understanding of my talents and deficiencies, personal strengths and weaknesses. Most importantly, I have an enhanced sense of what elements in a lifestyle and a career are important to me. The desire to create and synthesize in an intellectually challenging environment, with supportive and stimulating colleagues are among the most important of these elements. Even more important is my desire to work with those less fortunate than myself and give back out of what I have been given. Medical school will present many new challenges and opportunities for learning, maturing, and more specifically defining my goals. Despite the changes and variations I am sure to undergo, I know the theme will still resonate.

Strengths

This is a unique applicant whose background and experiences will add diversity to the incoming class. She is aware of this and capitalizes on it in her essay. Through her experiences, she presents herself as an interesting, competent, and focused individual.

Weaknesses

Though this is a strong essay, the analogies to music and musical performances are overdone.

ESSAY 33: Survivor of Anorexia; Emergency Medical Technician Training; Clinic Experience; Medical Volunteer in Honduras; HIV Test Counselor

Accepted at: Stanford University School of Medicine; Duke University School of Medicine; Tufts University School of Medicine; Harvard Medical School; Mount Sinai School of Medicine, CUNY; Albert Einstein College of Medicine, Yeshiva University

I decided that I wanted to be a doctor sometime after my four month incarceration in Columbia Presbyterian Children's Hospital, as I struggled with anorexia nervosa. Through the maturation process that marked my recovery, I slowly came to realize that my pediatrician had saved my life—despite my valiant efforts to the contrary. Out of our individual stubborn wills was born a kind of mutual respect, and he is one of the people who make up my small collection of heroes.

I admire doctors who understand both what is said and what is held back, who move comfortably around the world of the body, and who treat all patients with respect. I am lucky because a few of them have become my impromptu teachers, taking a little extra time to instruct me in anatomy, disease or courtesy. During my Emergency Medical Technician training, one of the emergency room doctors took me to radiology to point out the shadow of a fracture in a CT-scan and trusted me to hold a little girl's lip while he inserted sutures. The physicians in the Hospital 12 de Octubre in Madrid, Spain taught me to hear lung sounds and to feel an enlarged liver and spleen. They explained the social and medical difficulties associated with the management of pediatric AIDS until I understood the Spanish well enough to begin asking questions; then they answered them.

I work now in the Mayfield Community Clinic, which provides primary care to members of the Spanish-speaking community near Stanford University. My job as a patient advocate involves taking histories, performing simple procedures and providing family planning and HIV counseling.

I try to use the knowledge I have gained from class and practice to formulate the right set of questions to ask each patient, but I am constantly reminded of how much I have to learn. I look at a baby and notice its cute, pudgy toes. Dr. V. plays with it while conversing with its mother, and in less than a minute has noted its responsiveness, strength, and attachment to its parent, and checked its reflexes, color and hydration. Gingerly, I search for the tympanic membrane in the ears of a cooperative child and touch an infant's warm, soft belly, willing my hands to have a measure of Dr. V.'s competence.

I first felt the need to be competent regarding the human body when I volunteered with the Amigos de Las Americas program in the town of T. in Lempira, Honduras. The hospital available to the people of T. (at a day's ride in the bed of a truck) was "where one went to die," so my partner and I, with our basic first aid certifications and our $15 Johnson & Johnson kits, quickly became makeshift "doctors." The responsibility initially created a heady feeling; a distressed mother called on us to bandage the toe her eight-year-old son had accidentally sliced to the bone with his machete. I told him the story of Beauty and the Beast in broken Spanish while my partner and I soaked the dirt from his toe, and during the following week we watched him heal.

Then our foster-mother, who normally tended to the sick, told my partner and me to "check on the foot" of D. The gentle-eyed, sixty-five year old man lay on his bed, his leg encased in bloody bandages from mid-calf to toe. After performing surgery, the hospital had given him a bottle of injectable antibiotics and some clean needles and sent him home without bandages or further instructions. My partner and I had not been trained to handle so serious a situation. We did not know what had happened; we did not know what the antibiotics were (or if they were actually antibiotics); we did not know if handling D.'s blood put us at risk for disease. We wanted to leave, but leaving the house meant leaving D. and betraying our foster-mother's trust. So we injected the antibiotics and cleaned and bandaged the wound every day for our remaining two weeks in Honduras although we felt ill-equipped for the responsibility, crippled by our ignorance and lack of supplies.

In T., I did not feel qualified to receive the trust the townspeople gave so willingly. As an HIV-antibody test counselor in California, I struggle everyday to win my clients' confidence. Somehow a twenty-one-year-old, Caucasian female must be sincere, knowledgeable and open enough to earn the respect of a fifty-five-year-old man who could be her father, a high school sophomore, an ex-drug addict, and a pregnant Latina woman. My clients are black, white, straight, gay, Ph.D. candidates and illiterate; some choose to come to me while others have court-orders. Yet to communicate effectively, each client must have enough confidence in me to engage in dialogue about his drug or sex life and to believe what I tell him, whether or not he chooses to act on our discussion.

Speaking with patients, doctors and community members has opened my eyes to some of the difficulties involved with healthcare provision, and I hope I have given some inspiration or comfort in exchange for the knowledge I have received. I want these lessons in openness and compassion to shape my understanding of medicine and allow me to become the type of doctor I admire.

Strengths

This is a great essay. It is personal, interesting, and full of relevant experience. It leaves out mention of virtually anything that could be found in the application and focuses on the soft skills that the admissions committee might not otherwise learn about the applicant. It is well written and entertaining to read.

Weaknesses

None.

ESSAY 34: Hospital Observer; Attempt to Save a Life Using CPR; Elder in the Church of Jesus Christ of Latter-day Saints
Accepted at: Harvard Medical School

Most of the understanding that I have gained of the importance of medicine in my life has been acquired experientially. To be sure, the scientific aspects of the field attract and stimulate me, but the motivation to forsake other intellectually stimulating endeavors has come from things I have felt and seen, not texts I have read and analyzed. Many of the insights I have gained have come through observing committed health care providers; some have come through providing help myself.

I have spent many hours with various physicians who have graciously invited me to shadow them in a day's work. One experience was particularly powerful for me. An old friend of the family, a pediatrician, related to me that he once submitted to the vocational aptitude tests administered by his college's office of career services. The results indicated he should be a minister. He was chagrined, as he related that his church has no paid ministry, but he quite eloquently explained to me the ways that a sensitive physician can fill that role, without a particular theological slant. As I watched him interact with his patients affectionately, but always appropriately, I was excited to observe that his comments were not merely rhetoric. His patients felt his concern and support, and I was inspired to adjust my understanding of the deportment of an effective physician. I want to treat my patients the way Dr. Durham treats his.

Another important insight about medicine I gained from a rather dramatic night aboard the Moscow-St. Petersburg express train. As I was attempting to get cozy in my compartment, a rather frantic voice echoed throughout the corridor, "Kto-nibud' vrach?" Assuming that I was as close as they'd come to a doctor (I had, by then, spent nearly two months in their medical system), I got up and identified myself as someone potentially helpful. The fellow, an engineer on the train, led me in a race down the long train which to me, in its own strange way, was reminiscent of a chase scene in a James Bond film. We finally arrived at a cabin, where a group of very frightened Spanish tourists had gathered. Praying that my Spanish would suffice, I began CPR on a member of their group whose heart had suddenly stopped beating. I taught his friends the rudiments of CPR in my broken Spanish, and we began a process doomed to failure from its beginning. I discovered later that he had been dead for 15 min. when I arrived. As sad as I am that he died, as sympathetic as I am to his family, I am grateful for the things I learned from that experience about compassion and the appropriate spirit of medicine. As we took turns with chest compression and artificial ventilation, I watched two of his friends perform the emergency procedure in a way that almost seemed a religious ritual. Their minds were focused, their attention reserved solely for their friend. They counted the beats with an amazing precision, correcting me when my rhythm became irregular by less than a second. Their mouths were poised to deliver a kiss of life at each repetition of the word "cinco." This process continued for two-and-a-half hours. I simply could not bear to tell his weeping wife that the situation was hopeless, and I felt very much overwhelmed by the majesty of his friends, never stopping for a moment to consider their aching arms. The first thing that struck me was the sense of self-forgetful devotion. That image has not left me in the year that has followed. The second was the absolute necessity of attention to detail. Their perfect commitment to exact detail inspired me to be more meticulous in critical situations. A father and husband died, and I hope that the lessons I learned from that experience, as I apply them in medicine, will be a suitable memorial to him.

Finally, I have learned much from serving in the Church of Jesus Christ of Latter-day Saints. As an Elder in the Church, I have frequently been called to hospitals to comfort, aid, and administer to members who are ill. I've lost count of the number of times I've visited people at home and in the hospital, but I have gained a very clear sense of what it means to comfort, to empathize, to provide strength. Perhaps my most sacred memory in this regard is a quiet farewell to my father, who died of complications associated with diabetes. There, in a sterile, uninviting hospital room, lay my father, pale and pained, but peaceful. We talked intimately for about an hour, fully aware that he would be dead within the week. Although, quite frankly, I was overcome with emotion at the time, I have since thought about the change that experience has wrought in my understanding of sick people that I visit. I have a much fuller sense that each patient is someone's beloved father, someone's close friend, someone's dear sister. I would hope that my father would take great pleasure in knowing that I treated my patients with sincere love and concern, the kind I proffered him.

Ultimately, as wonderful a scientific opportunity as medicine is, as great the chances to stretch the very limits of my cognitive capacity, it draws me with people. Time spent with them, grappling with their fears and ailments, have shaped me and strengthened me. I hope to repay that, to be true to the examples that have been provided me.

Strengths

This is a powerful essay. It is written with such emotion that it invokes emotion in its reader as well. It is personal, engaging, and memorable. Much can be ascertained about the applicant through his experiences and his words. Once again, this is an applicant who has focused his discussions on topics not found in his application. The effectiveness of this approach cannot be stressed enough. It allows the applicant to present much more of himself to the admissions committee, and thus much more to draw the committee to him.

Weaknesses

There were a few grammatical issues that should have been resolved before the essay was submitted.

ESSAY 35: Career Switcher from Veterinarian Technician; Emergency Medical Technician; Parents' Influence
Accepted at: Washington University School of Medicine; George Washington University School of Medicine; Harvard Medical School; University of Massachusetts Medical School; University of Maryland School of Medicine

She dropped the box on the table and left the room because she didn't want to watch. I could understand her feelings: many of our clients at the veterinary clinic chose not to observe the distressing moment when life slipped away from their pet. Still, I always felt for the animals whose owners couldn't face the reality of the decision they'd made, animals who would die surrounded by relative strangers.

As I waited for the veterinarian to come perform the euthanasia, I stroked the dehydrated cat's bony back. She lay still, tired from fighting the sickness. My petting her seemed a necessity: the only way to provide one final pleasure for this old animal. She barely responded, maybe a slight twitch of the whiskers. But then, just before the vet stepped into the room, my little patient started to purr. It began softly but grew to a warm rumble, filling the room with the sound of a cat's contentedness. I had, happily, made this cat as comfortable as was possible. She kept on purring even as I held her and the doctor injected the thick pink solution into her vein. The sound faded quietly as her body went limp in my arms.

As a veterinary technician, I don't think I could have asked for a better introduction to the power of medicine. At the clinic I experienced first hand the day-to-day life of medical practice. We treated outpatient and boarding animals who were essentially healthy: administering vaccines, drawing blood, giving daily medications and offering general medical advice. I performed lab tests and maintain hospital supplies. We also cared for animals whose conditions were critical: I noted their progress, reported to the doctor, and carried out his orders for treatment. Therapies included special feeding, intravenous or subcutaneous fluid administration, and medications of all kinds. This intensive care afforded me the chance to observe diagnostic techniques and the decisions for treatments that were based on the diagnoses. I also assisted during surgery, monitoring the vital signs of the patient using only a stethoscope, the air bag and my intuition for what was normal. I performed the pre- and post-operative duties and any treatments that were more easily done while the animals were sedated, such as thorough dental cleaning. I was therefore able to see the excitement of surgery and the satisfaction of using one's hands to directly heal a body.

Over those 2 years, I decided that I wanted to apply to medical school rather than veterinary school. I gradually found myself feeling out of touch with a large part of humanity. I realized that the pleasure of healing would be greater for me if the patients were people. This realization has been affirmed in my recent experiences shadowing doctors and training as a medical assistant. I feel there are greater challenges involved in caring for human beings: Treatment of critical illness in animals halts before human care does, since euthanasia is a readily available option for veterinarians. Human medicine therefore goes beyond most animal care, delving deeper to fight disease. In addition, there is a psychological dimension to human medicine that attracts me. Of course, interaction with patients is richer; I value and hope to encourage the contributions that patients make to their own well-being and health care. The true causes of healing and the role of the mind in restoring and maintaining the body are subjects that I find extremely compelling.

My training and experiences with medicine have contributed to how I envision myself practicing it. I greatly enjoyed the diversity of medicine practiced at the vet clinic; for this and other reasons I lean towards primary care or emergency medicine. In order to explore the latter option I am pursuing certification as an Emergency Medical Technician. I also appreciate the individual nature of service provided by a small, modest clinic, and would like to provide such personal care for the people I treat. I look forward to getting to know my patients as well as we at the clinic knew our clients and their pets.

I realize in retrospect that as a young girl I always assumed I would be a doctor. My father was a psychiatrist, and my mother entered medical school when I entered kindergarten. My mother provides a role model I still look to for guidance. Throughout my high school years and into my first year at college, I pursued activities in the medical sciences, such as advanced courses and a summer research assistant job at N.I.H. Although I began college as a pre-medical student, the wider options presented to me at school made me eager to explore other disciplines. I turned away from science during my undergraduate years, but am confident that my Swarthmore education will be invaluable in my development as a well-rounded physician. My experiences in medicine, healing the sick, comforting the ill and dying, and even the routine aspects of the work, hold a power for me that I cannot ignore. Since arriving at this decision and acting on it, I feel that I have come full circle. I have ended up in many ways where I began, but with far more experience. This is exactly where I want to be.

Student Comments

I don't think my essay was crucial in my acceptance, as my MCAT scores were very good, and my grades good. As well, I had worked and lived a while before applying, which broadened my experiences.

One tip on applying in general: Talk to 3rd and 4th years, and listen to what they say. They know more about medical school in general, and theirs in particular. Also, the clinical years really are more important than years 1 and 2. Look at what the clinical experience will be like in judging which school you want.

Strengths

This candidate brings a unique background to the applicant pool. While the role of veterinary technician might not typically stand out as good preparation for medical school, the applicant effectively describes her learning experience as one that seems to have prepared her quite well for her role as a future caregiver—whether to humans or animals. The applicant began the essay with an engaging story and her strong writing skills allowed her to hold the interest of the reader for the essay's entirety.

Weaknesses

Except for a typo in the third paragraph, the essay had no real weaknesses.

ESSAY 36: Environmental Study in Africa; Cancer Center Intern; Art History Background; Community Service; Literacy Volunteer
Accepted at: Cornell University Medical College

"Why on Earth do you want to study in Africa?" is a question I remember being asked frequently before I went to Kenya for the Dartmouth College Environmental Studies Program. At the time, I thought the question was absurd—I could not understand why anyone would not jump at the opportunity to live among and learn about such diverse and exciting peoples. However, after my three months of study throughout Kenya, I realized that not everyone could endure, much less enjoy, the experiences I had. For some people, the pit latrines, absence of running water, malarial mosquitoes and mud-dung huts would have defined the experience. For me, it was so much more: My time in Kenya was shaped by the Samburu pastoralists that shared their homes with us for a week, by the wild animals that we studied for hours on end, by the Kamba agriculturists that gave us a glimpse of their lifestyle over a weekend homestay, and by my Luo family in Nairobi. Indeed, my sojourns in Kenya would not have been enjoyed by everyone. But they were the profoundly educational and humanitarian experiences on which I thrive.

A career in medicine appears to be a lot like studying in Kenya. It is challenging, intense, filled with hard work, and extremely rewarding—but not for everyone. Many people cannot see beyond the years of demanding course work, sleep deprivation, and long work hours that are associated with the study and practice of medicine. Although these are realities of a physician's life, they are not what define it for me. A career as a physician excites me because it would allow me to further understand the fascinating science that dictates human life, and more importantly, it would allow me to work closely with people, while trying to understand and alleviate their suffering. My love for learning and passion for helping people drove me to Kenya, and they also fuel my desire to become a physician.

My first encounter with medical science was as a Women in Science Project Intern in the Norris Cotton Cancer Center of the

Dartmouth-Hitchcock Medical Center. I worked in the radiobiology lab of Dr. J., and was given the task of designing and carrying out experiments to measure the absorption and scattering coefficients of laser light in tissue-simulating media, for use in the development of Photodynamic Therapy (PDT) as a cancer treatment. The project was so exciting to me that it developed into a full-time summer position, which culminated in my contribution to a scientific paper, currently being reviewed by several journals for publication. My interest in the projects of Dr. O's laboratory was so substantial that I continued to work with her after the completion of the PDT project for over a year. Specifically, I assisted with experiments to correlate the rate of blood flow and the partial pressure of oxygen in tumors. My work resulted in a contribution to another abstract, submitted to the Regional Conference on Cancer Research at the UVM Cancer Center in Burlington, Vermont.

In addition to my enthusiasm for science, I have a deep-rooted interest in art history. My curiosity about the subject was sparked in high school; and by the time I graduated, it had become one of my favorite subjects. My interest continued through college and culminated in three months of study in Florence, Italy, with the Dartmouth College Art History Program. I hope to continue my study of art history throughout my life. Artistic interpretation is a good balance for data analysis and scientific exploration; it provides insight into an entirely different way of viewing the world.

However, both my research experiences and my study of art have left me devoid of the satisfaction of helping people that I have felt throughout high school and college, working directly with several community service organizations. When I was fifteen, I volunteered at a local hospital. Although I had few responsibilities, it was the first time I had interacted with patients. The satisfaction I derived from assisting these people solidified my desire to help others. That same summer, I traveled with several other students to Middlebury, Vermont to repair a homeless shelter. Later in high school, I became a member of Literacy Volunteers of America and tutored adult students in a local adult education center. Throughout my college career, I have been involved with Dartmouth's Students Fighting Hunger chapter. Few things in my college career have been as rewarding as working to help feed the people of the Upper Valley region through community awareness programs, fund-raising projects, and direct assistance in soup kitchens. Seeking to learn about the union of science and compassion in medical practice, I am spending part of this summer as a Student Observer in the Memorial Sloan-Kettering Cancer Center, Department of Thoracic Surgery. One of my highest priorities is to remain involved in humanitarian assistance throughout my life. The medical field would provide an ideal setting for me to fulfill this goal.

A career as a physician would unite my excitement for learning and my desire for helping others into a distinct whole. My life so far has been filled with many diverse experiences, teaching me much about both my own interest and the way in which I can best serve humanity. I look forward to integrating my interests and talents into a four-year medical education, and a lifelong medical career.

Strengths

Overall, this essay is good. Through her writing, the applicant presents herself as a well-rounded and interesting candidate. She seems driven by her humanitarian efforts, which lend credence to her claim of wanting a medical degree so that she can continue to help people. She presents her research projects in an interesting manner and her resulting accolades are impressive.

Weaknesses

The second paragraph could have been eliminated because the point that she wants to help people is stressed elsewhere and this paragraph added nothing substantial to the essay. The sixth paragraph reads too much like a list because she has included a lot of experiences but has not provided much substance for any of them.

ESSAY 37: Chapter Director at Habitat for Humanity; Author of Book on Third-World Medicine; Summer Research Intern
Accepted at: Cornell University Medical College

On the corner of 168th Street and Broadway in New York City there always seems to be a line of people. They begin waiting as early as 6:30 A.M., so by the time I arrive for work at eight, the line has over 150 people on it stretching around the block and extending a good fifth of a mile down Broadway. It was during my Summer Research Internship at Columbia Presbyterian Medical Center that I first understood how becoming a physician would enable me to make that line for their urban clinic move faster.

By lunch-time the line dwindles a little; people occupy their time listening to iPods, reading newspapers, second guessing the New York Yankees starting lineup and calming down children restless from standing still for several hours. Perhaps one day the ramifications of the research I had only begun on the uptake rates of iron might improve the nutrition of those on line. The thought that I could be doing something to help, if only I had the medical expertise like both my parents, rages through my brain like the sound of the red "A" train many of the patients took to get here.

Watching them, I realize that when I become a physician I will be empowered to make that line move faster and subtly change the world. Following my three years as the Project Director of the campus chapter of Habitat for Humanity—renovating condemned housing for underprivileged families—I have been able to experience this feeling. Our group of volunteers, which had no prior knowledge of construction or architecture, learned enough construction and urban planning to rebuild a condemned 120-year-old house for the seven-member Losado family.

During this process, we have "healed" a house, but, more importantly, we have revitalized a community. Just as when a physician alleviates his patients' suffering, he or she "heals" the patients' family. Neighbors had rallied behind our efforts by providing us with nourishment while we worked. They began to know one another and even formed a neighborhood watch to protect their renovated community. Encouraged by our initial accomplishment, we will be working on a row of six townhouses. Leaving that construction site better than we found it epitomizes my desire to serve through medicine. Being a doctor will allow me to do the same, whether on 168th Street or in similar clinics any place in the world.

On a recent trip to India I toured the decrepit urban clinic facilities at Baroda Medical College—my father's alma mater—and the need to help became ever stronger. While crossing the school's open courtyard, I saw a patient with a large mass protruding from her neck. Noticing my alarm, my father pointed out how easily this patient's goiter could have been treated. Though my basic and clinical research training thus far have not yet equipped me to heal her condition, I donated my current skills at that clinic, setting up a computer database of cases to supplant their outmoded methods of medical record-keeping.

My experience helped me to write a first-hand account of third-world medicine for my third book, The Shower Song Groove, so that others will know and be inspired to contribute and help remediate these appalling conditions. When I returned to school, I used the writing skills I sharpened as a writer and editor of The Daily Princetonian to share what I had seen with my peers in "Prescriptions"—my bi-weekly editorial column. India's medical problems are not too far away from the long lines on the corner of Broadway and 168th Street.

By 7 P.M., I leave the building and turn the corner to wait for my bus home. The line has few people on it, as many have abandoned hope of seeing a physician today. They pledge to be in line earlier tomorrow. The sight of disheartened men and women, heads down, turning toward the subway station reminds me of a discussion I had with the late tennis star, Arthur Ashe, whom I interviewed for The Daily Princetonian only months before his death. He asked me about my career plans and when I told him that I wanted to become a physician, he shared with me his view of great medical care. "Truly great medicine is not the urge to surpass others at all cost, but the urge to serve others at all cost." That must be my motto as I make the line on 168th Street move a little faster.

Strengths

This is a strong essay because it is personal and interesting. The applicant showcases his relevant medical experience through his stories. He also reveals his motivation to help others through his work with Habitat for Humanity. He does not focus on areas that can be found elsewhere in his application. He took advantage of the opportunity to unveil his softer side to the admissions committee, affording them the chance to see him as a person and not just another MCAT score.

Weaknesses

None.

ESSAY 38: Rower
Accepted to: Cornell University Medical College

"Power ten, next stroke!" shouts the coxswain over the speaker system. We rush past English countryside as our rowing shell skims along the River Cam. "One—drive it hard! Two!. . . Three!. . ." Each rower in the eight quietly focuses on his own stroke, not communicating with anyone. In the midst of the physical exertion of taking stroke after stroke, I am amazed by what I am doing and where I am doing it.

I chose to go to Cambridge for a year abroad because I thought a year in England would add a new dimension to my education, both culturally and academically. New York is always stimulating, but I wanted to experience life somewhere else. I intuitively knew that a change of perspective would be rewarding. I was determined to continue my scientific studies, and Cambridge offers some of the best academic science in the world. I was excited to have been awarded a place in the university. Happily, I found an activity which enabled me to both immerse myself in English culture and achieve a sense of personal accomplishment. That activity was rowing.

I chose to row for several reasons. Rowing provided an effective way to meet many people and assimilate into English life. I turned down an offer to join the Cambridge sailing team because I felt that rowing would better introduce me to English culture. Sailing for another year would have been the predictable, safe option; I wanted a new challenge. Rowing was Cambridge's most popular and traditional sport. I was eager to learn new customs and acquire a mastery over a new skill. In addition, disciplined exercise has always helped me to focus on important things in my life, like doing school work or deciding to go to medical school.

Never having rowed before, I had to start from the bottom, in a novice boat. Practice commenced before sunrise, and we had to run down to the boathouse each morning because, as we were told, every rower going back over a hundred years had had to do it. We practiced in leaky, old wooden boats that had their heyday back in the 50's. Yelling commands through dented-in megaphones, sixty-year-old coaches dressed in tweed followed us along the bank in bicycles older than they were.

The richness of the English rowing tradition inspired me. The boat-house was strewn with historic championship awards bearing inscriptions from places as far away as communist Russia and as near as prestigious Henley. While my boat did not contribute to the grand collection, I did have the satisfaction of upholding the tradition and high standard of rowing in England by being a participant.

After much improvement, I was promoted to the college's second boat by the second term. The second boat required much more commitment to training. I had never been in so fit and focused before in my life. It was a challenge to maintain such a high level of performance, but my diligence paid dividends as we placed among the top boats in our regattas.

One of my goals while abroad had been to travel around England, using Cambridge as a starting point for journeys to various towns and cities. My plans were curtailed because rowing required so much of my time, and I was determined to finish what I had started and to see my commitment through. I discovered that rowing on a short stretch of the Cam enriched my education more than any traveling could do.

Strengths

The applicant reveals something personal about himself by discussing his experience abroad and his participation on the rowing team. He discusses experiences that would not be found anywhere else on his application.

Weaknesses

Though it is advisable to discuss experiences outside of what can be found on the application, this applicant never ties the experience into his motivation to pursue medicine. He altogether avoids the topics of his motivation, his goals, and any relevant experience that might make him a strong candidate. The essay seems to have been thrown together quickly and could have benefited from outside feedback. The applicant most likely had very strong credentials and felt comfortable stepping outside of the usual parameters of the application essay.

Essay Index

EXPERIENCE

Hospital and Research Experience	5, 7, 9, 11, 14, 16, 20, 22, 23, 24, 27, 29
Hospital/clinic experience only	2, 12, 15, 17, 21, 28, 33, 34
Research experience only	3, 4, 6, 25, 26, 36
Volunteers	4, 7, 8, 9, 10, 15, 16, 19, 21, 27, 33, 37
Teachers, Tutors, Advisors, Counselors	4, 5, 6, 8, 12, 14, 20, 22, 24, 28, 36

EDUCATIONAL BACKGROUNDS

General Liberal Arts	7, 12, 18
Literature	1, 11
Theater	7
Military	2
Art History	28, 36
Math	17
Music	32
Psychology	32
Classics	22
Asian Studies	12
Archeology	30
Engineering	9, 14

INTERNATIONAL/CULTURAL EXPERIENCE

Haiti	19
Brazil	21
Iceland and Paris	28
Hungary and Estonia	31
Indonesia	32
Honduras	33
Africa	36
India	37

CAREER SWITCHERS

From business	3, 21
From engineer	9, 14
From broadcasting/communication	18
Public health	19
Veterinarian	35

MOTIVATION

From childhood	4, 5, 10, 12, 13, 24, 29
Latecomers	21, 22
Physicians in family	5, 12, 22, 24, 29, 35
Personal experience with illness/ accidents	2, 15, 16, 27, 33, 34
Unpleasant medical/doctor experience	10

OTHER

Religious	6, 13, 34
Writers	14, 32, 37
Athletes	10, 27, 38
Musicians	6, 10, 11, 32

Index

A

Accomplishments, 23
Action lead, 53–54
Active voice, 60
Admissions committee, 11–19
Admissions officers, 10–11, 68
AMCAS. *See* American Medical College
    Application Service
American Medical College Application Service,
    3–4, 81–167
Application, 5, 67, 72–73
Applying, 1–6
Audience, 9–19

B

Background, 76
Brainstorming, 20

C

Character, 76–77
Chronological assessments, 23
Chronological structure, 46–48
Clinical experience, 35
Close, 55–56
Commas, 51
Communication skills, 12, 14
Compare/contrast, 46
Conclusion, 55–56
Creative lead, 53
Creative writing exercises, 21–22

D

Details, 15–16
Dialogue lead, 55
Diversity, 32–33

E

English majors, 33
Essay writing
    alternative approaches, 39
    audience, 9–19
    details used in, 15–16
    exercises in, 21–22
    honesty in, 16–17
    personal element in, 14–15
    preparation for, 7–8
    telling a story in, 16
Ethics, 76–77
Etiquette, 69–70
Examples, 21
Excuses, 37–38
Experiences, 35–36, 74–75

F

Faculty interviewer, 79
Feedback, 19, 61
Fees, 5–6
Free-flow writing, 22

G

Gimmicks, 17–18
Goals, 24–25
GPA, 2, 10

H

Honesty, 16–17, 69
Hospital experience, 35

I

Illegal questions, 77
Informative lead, 55
Inspiration, 21
International experience, 34
Interview
    description of, 5, 63
    preparing for, 65–70
    tips for, 66–69
    types of, 66
Interviewer, 67, 79
Interview questions, 72–79
Introductions, 52
Inventory, 21–22

J

Journal writing, 22

L

Language abilities, 12
Lead, 52–55
Letters of recommendation, 4–5

M

Materials, 20–25
MCAT. *See* Medical College Admission
    Test
Mechanical errors, 18–19
Medical College Admission Test, 2–3
Medical field, 75–76
Medical issues, 38–39
Medical schools
    applying to, 1–6
    curriculum of, 2
    personal statements for, 36–37
Motivation, 11–12, 29, 73–74
Musical abilities, 32

N
Narrative, 48–49, 58

O
Open-ended questions, 73
Outline, 44–48
Overpreparedness, 71

P
Paragraphs, 49–50
Passive voice, 60
Personal, 14–15
Personality, 24, 76
Personal lead, 54
Personal questions, 77
Personal statements, 26–39, 81–167
Plagiarizing, 81
Pre-med courses, 2
Proofreading, 18, 60–61

Q
Qualifications, 35–36, 74–75
Quotation lead, 54–55

R
Reading out loud, 61
Redundancies, 37
Relaxation, 68
Religion, 34
Research experience, 35
Revealing lead, 54
Revision, 57–59
Rough spots, 78

S
Secondary applications, 5
Self-assessments, 23–25

Semicolons, 51
Sentences, 51–52
Sincerity, 73–74
Skills, 12–13, 23–24
Soft skills, 12–13, 63
Standard lead, 53
Standard structure, 44–46
Stream of consciousness, 22
Structure
    chronological, 46–48
    compare/contrast, 46
    reviewing of, 58–59
    standard, 44–46
Student interviewer, 79
Substance, 58

T
Telling a story, 16
Thank-you notes, 70
Themes, 27–39
Thesaurus, 50–51
Transcripts, 4
Transitions, 50

U
Underpreparation, 71
Uniqueness, 31–34

V
Verbs, 51

W
Words, 50–51
Writing skills, 12

Is medical school in your future? This book gives you a head start

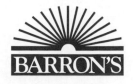

The hardest obstacle to overcome in becoming a physician is getting admitted to a medical school. This book cuts through the official jargon and tells you exactly what you really need to do to be accepted. For instance, how to choose a college and a major field of study, how to avoid the "Premed Syndrome," how to cope with the MCAT, when, where, and how to apply to medical school, and how to deal with rejections. With a directory of AMA-approved medical schools.

Reviews from previous editions:

"Majoring in non-science will probably raise your overall GPA and put you in a more advantageous position when seeking admission..."

"Apart from their annual pilgrimage to a medical school (a trip which you can more profitably make on your own), the value of [premedical clubs] is dubious..."

"The premedical adviser holds no degree or certification for the job, is not licensed, and is not subject to peer review. The adviser is only as good as personal interest and involvement allow."

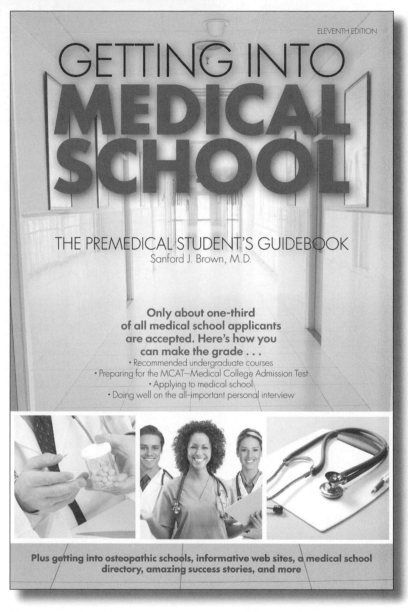

Paperback, ISBN: 978-0-7641-4597-1, $14.99, *Can$17.99*

Barron's Educational Series, Inc.
250 Wireless Blvd.
Hauppauge, N.Y. 11788
Order toll-free: 1-800-645-3476
Order by fax: 1-631-434-3217

In Canada:
Georgetown Book Warehouse
34 Armstrong Ave.
Georgetown, Ontario L7G 4R9
Canadian orders: 1-800-247-7160
Order by fax: 1-800-887-1594

Prices subject to change without notice.

——— To order ———
Available at your local book store
or visit **www.barronseduc.com**

(#37) R 11/11

GETTING INTO MEDICAL OR DENTAL SCHOOL IS TOUGH!

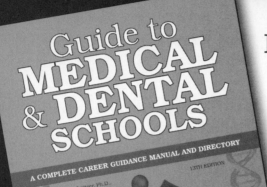

Here's the book that will increase your chances . . .

Guide to Medical and Dental Schools, 13th Edition

by Dr. Saul Wischnitzer, with Edith Wischnitzer

It's a comprehensive school directory—and a lot more! You'll find detailed guidance and advice on all phases of the medical and dental school application and training processes, including . . .

- Examples of typical forms to fill out
- A description of modern medical education
- A self-assessment admission profile
- A model Medical College Admission Test, as well as Dental Admission Test questions, all with answers

You'll also find profiles of all AMA, AOA, and ADA accredited medical, osteopathic, and dental schools throughout the United States and Canada, with information on admission requirements, course requirements, filing deadlines, tuition and fees, and much more.

ISBN 978-0-7641-4752-4
$18.99, Can$21.99

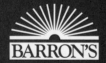

Barron's Educational Series, Inc.
250 Wireless Blvd.
Hauppauge, N.Y. 11788
Order toll-free: 1-800-645-3476
Order by fax: 1-631-434-3217

In Canada:
Georgetown Book Warehouse
34 Armstrong Ave.
Georgetown, Ontario L7G 4R9
Canadian orders:
1-800-247-7160
Order by fax: 1-800-887-1594

To order visit us at **www.barronseduc.com** or your local book store

Prices subject to change without notice.

(#92) R 10/11

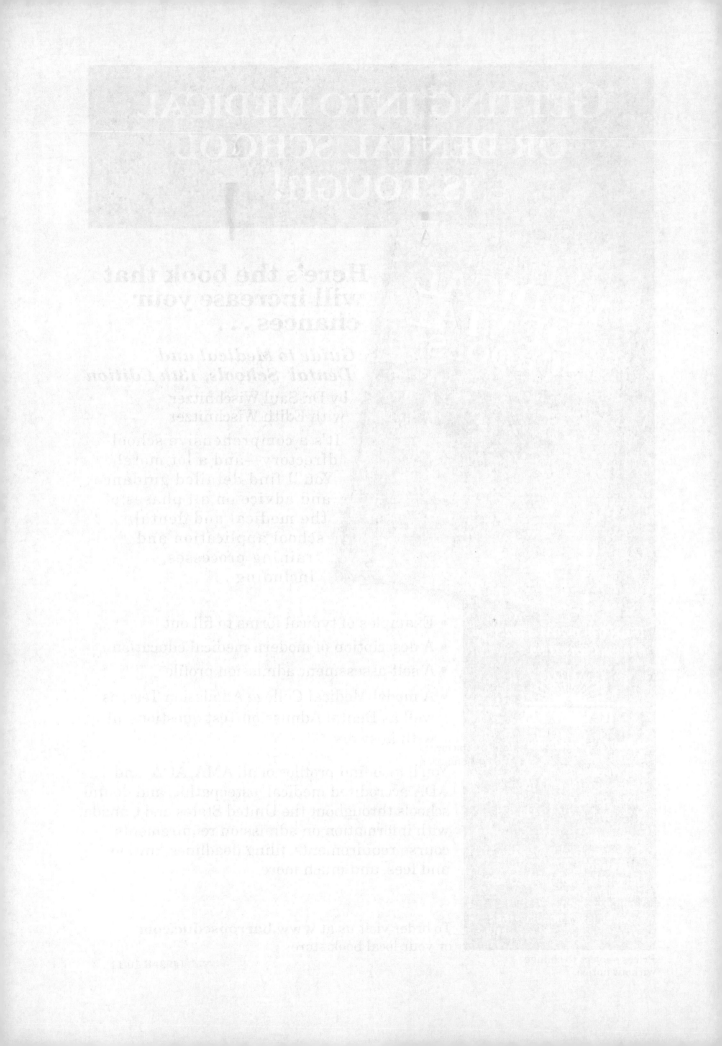

Improved grades in anatomy and physiology courses start with this selection of BARRON'S titles

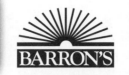

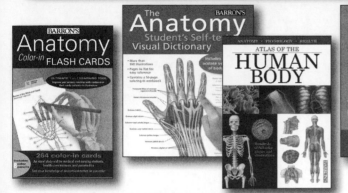

Anatomy Color-in Flash Cards
Kurt Albertine, Ph.D.; Edited by Ken Ashwell, Ph.D.
A unique set of boxed flash cards combines two study tools into one package. By coloring the anatomically correct illustrations, students are more likely to remember shapes and features.
Boxed Set, 978-0-7641-9677-5, $28.99, *Can$34.50*

The Anatomy Student's Self-Test Visual Dictionary
Ken Ashwell, Ph.D.
A workbook section focuses on the body's muscle and skeletal systems, and eight color acetate overlay sheets illustrate body systems.
Paperback: 978-0-7641-4724-1, $29.99, *Can$34.50*

The Anatomy Student's Self-Test Coloring Book
Kurt Albertine, Ph.D.
Anatomically accurate line art shows body parts. Readers can shade them in with colored pencils. Overlay sheets illustrate the body's muscles, bones, and organs.
Paperback: 978-0-7641-3777-8, $24.99, *Can$29.99*

Atlas of the Human Body
Adolfo Cassan
Scientifically accurate full-color illustrations complement clear, correct explanations of the body's organs and their functions.
Hardcover, 978-0-7641-6091-2, $24.99, *Can$29.99*

Barron's Anatomy Flash Cards, 2nd Ed.
Kurt Albertine, Ph.D.
A set of flash cards showing muscles, bones, and organs are color coded according to their general body functions.
Boxed Set, 978-0-7641-6159-9, $26.99, *Can$32.50*

Barron's Educational Series, Inc.
250 Wireless Blvd.
Hauppauge, N.Y. 11788
Call toll-free: 1-800-645-3476

In Canada:
Georgetown Book Warehouse
34 Armstrong Ave.
Georgetown, Ontario L7G 4R9
Call toll-free: 1-800-247-7160

Essential Atlas of Anatomy
Parramón Studios
The human body is shown in detailed, scientifically correct full-color illustrations. Fifteen separate sections examine both male and female bodies. Here is a handy home reference, as well as a fine supplement to classroom science textbooks.
Paperback, 978-0-7641-1833-3, $13.99, *Can$16.99*

Essential Atlas of Physiology
Parramón Studios
This information-packed atlas combines color photos, diagrams, and illustrations with lucid text to describe the human body and its functions. Following a general introduction, separate spreads focus on all major physiology topics.
Paperback, 978-0-7641-3093-9, $14.99, *Can$16.99*

Dictionary of Medical Terms, 6th Ed.
Mikel A. Rothenberg, M.D., Charles F. Chapman, and Rebecca Sell, M.D.
Thousands of terms and definitions cover diseases and their symptoms, human anatomy, medications, and much more. Includes line illustrations and extensive cross references.
Paperback, 978-0-7641-4758-6, $14.99, *Can$16.99*

E-Z Anatomy and Physiology, 2nd Ed.
E. Edward Alcamo, Ph.D., and Barbara Krumhardt, Ph.D.
This review of the human body's structural framework and functions is a self-teaching manual focused to improve students' grades. Its text, supplemented with charts, graphs, diagrams, and line art, reviews anatomy and physiology on a college-101 level.
Paperback, 978-0-7641-4468-4, $16.99, *Can$19.99*

The Student's Anatomy of Exercise Manual
Ken Ashwell, Ph.D.
Health trainers, and all who need to get into better physical shape, can profit from 50 essential exercises, described and illustrated, and supplemented with a workbook section to help readers understand the rationale behind each exercise. Color illustrations.
Paperback, 978-1-4380-0113-5, $24.99, *Can$28.50*

To order — Available at your local book store
or visit **www.barronseduc.com**

Prices subject to change without notice.

(191) R 5/12

Your first important step on the journey to medical school

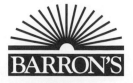

Barron's MCAT with CD-ROM

Jay Cutts, M.A., Executive Editor

Written by a team of specialists who train students for success on graduate school exams, this combination book and CD-ROM gives prospective medical students the three things they'll need most on exam day:

• Extensive subject review material for a solid understanding of all exam topics

• A critical set of time-management strategies to help students minimize stress and maximize their scores

• Test-taking practice in the form of a diagnostic test, four full-length model MCATs in the manual, and an enclosed CD-ROM with two more tests that closely reflect actual computer-based MCAT test-taking conditions. All questions are answered and explained.

The book's review chapters cover all MCAT test sections: Physical Sciences, Verbal Reasoning, the MCAT Essays, and Biological Sciences. Also featured is a multi-month study plan to prepare test takers for success when they take this all-important exam.

Paperback with CD-ROM, ISBN: 978-1-4380-7070-4
$49.99, *Can$56.99*

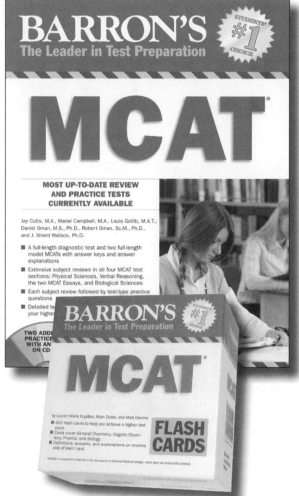

Barron's MCAT Flash Cards

Lauren Marie Kupillas, Brian Drolet, and Matt Giovine

Students preparing to take the Medical College Admission Test will value this set of flash cards as they brush up on questions typical of those that appear on the actual MCAT. The cards—with questions or concepts on the front and answers or concept explanations on the reverse side—are divided into four sections: General Chemistry, Organic Chemistry, Physics, and Biology. Cards measure 4 1/2" by 2 3/4", and have a hole in one corner to accommodate a metal key-ring style card holder that is included with the cards. The ring allows students to arrange the flash cards for study sessions in any sequence that suits their needs. These flash cards make excellent study aids when used alone, but are even more effective when used in tandem with Barron's MCAT test preparation manual.

Boxed set, 456 cards, ISBN: 978-0-7641-9692-8, $18.99, *Can$22.99*

Barron's Educational Series, Inc.
250 Wireless Blvd.
Hauppauge, N.Y. 11788
Order toll-free: 1-800-645-3476
Order by fax: 1-631-434-3217

In Canada:
Georgetown Book Warehouse
34 Armstrong Ave.
Georgetown, Ontario L7G 4R9
Canadian orders: 1-800-247-7160
Order by fax: 1-800-887-1594

——To order——
Available at your
local book store or visit
www.barronseduc.com

Prices subject to change without notice.

(#42) R9/11

Notes